Dental Basic Life Support

A Step-by-Step Handbook

Blessing Isaackson

Disclaimer

This handbook is for **learning and training purposes only**.

- It explains the principles of Dental Basic Life Support.
- It does **not replace professional training or certification**.
- Always follow local guidelines and ensure you have the proper skills before applying these steps.
- The author and publisher are not liable for misuse of the information.

Second Edition

Feedback: bisaackson@gmail.com
ISBN (eBook): 978-1-0683557-0-7
ISBN (Paperback): 978-1-0683557-1-4

Contents

Foreword

Medical emergencies in the dental setting are rare, but when they occur, they demand immediate, confident, and well-coordinated action. Dental professionals are often the first responders in these critical moments, and the ability to act swiftly and correctly can be life-saving. *Dental Basic Life Support: A Step-by-Step Handbook* has been developed by Blessing Isaackson to ensure every member of the dental team is equipped with the knowledge, skills, and confidence required to respond effectively.

At Fairview Training Ltd, we believe that high-quality education should be clear, practical, and directly applicable to real clinical environments. Training should empower learners, not overwhelm them. This handbook reflects our commitment to structured learning, visual clarity, and straightforward explanations that translate national clinical guidance into actionable steps within the dental practice.

The content is aligned with current **Resuscitation Council UK** and **NICE** guidance, alongside best practice from emergency care and dentistry. Each section has been carefully designed to support both comprehensive learning and rapid reference, making it suitable for students, newly qualified clinicians, and experienced professionals seeking to refresh or maintain their competence.

Our aim is to foster a culture of preparedness where medical emergencies are managed with calm, competence, and professionalism. Every patient deserves a dental team that is ready to act. Every clinician deserves training that builds confidence and capability. And every practice benefits from embedding emergency preparedness as a fundamental standard of care.

We commend your commitment to patient safety and continuous professional development, and we are proud to support you in delivering the highest standards of emergency care in dentistry.

Fairview Training Ltd

Aims of Basic Life Support

In line with Resuscitation Council UK (2025) and NICE guidance, Basic Life Support aims to:

- **Preserve life** — respond rapidly and effectively to prevent avoidable death.
- **Prevent deterioration** — identify early warning signs and intervene before the patient's condition worsens.
- **Promote recovery** — provide timely support and stabilisation until advanced medical help takes over.

Infection Control in the Dental Practice

Effective infection prevention and control (IPC) is fundamental to the delivery of safe, high-quality dental care. Dental teams routinely work in close proximity to patients' blood, saliva, and respiratory secretions, and frequently undertake aerosol-generating procedures (AGPs), all of which increase the risk of transmission of infectious agents. Robust IPC systems protect patients, staff, and the wider community and are a legal and professional requirement under the **Health and Social Care Act 2008**, **HTM 01-05**, and regulatory expectations of the **Care Quality Commission (CQC)**.[12]

1. Principles of Infection Transmission

Infection occurs when a sufficient number of pathogenic microorganisms enter a susceptible host via a recognised route of transmission. In the dental setting, the principal routes include:

- **Direct contact** with blood, saliva, or other body fluids
- **Indirect contact** via contaminated instruments, equipment, or environmental surfaces
- **Airborne and droplet transmission** from aerosols generated during dental procedures

Because a patient's infectious status cannot be reliably identified through history alone, **Standard Infection Control Precautions (SICPs)** must be applied to **all patients, at all times.**[3]

2. Standard Infection Control Precautions (SICPs)

SICPs form the foundation of IPC in dental practice and must be consistently applied across all clinical activities.

Hand Hygiene

- Hand hygiene is the **single most effective measure** for preventing cross-infection.[3]
- Alcohol-based hand rubs and antimicrobial liquid soap must be readily available at the point of care.
- Hands must be decontaminated **before and after each patient contact**, after glove removal, and after contact with bodily fluids or contaminated surfaces.

Personal Protective Equipment (PPE)

- Appropriate PPE includes **single-use gloves, fluid-resistant surgical masks or respirators (where indicated), eye/face protection, and clinical clothing**.
- PPE must be selected based on the level of risk and disposed of safely after use.
- Staff must be trained in correct **donning and doffing** techniques to avoid self-contamination.[4]

Respiratory Hygiene and Ventilation

- Patients should be encouraged to use tissues and perform hand hygiene when coughing or sneezing.
- Clinical areas must have **adequate ventilation**, with enhanced ventilation measures in place where AGPs are undertaken, in line with national guidance.[5]

3. Decontamination of Dental Instruments

All reusable instruments must be decontaminated in accordance with **HTM 01-05**, essential or best-practice standards.[2]

Cleaning

- Manual cleaning should be avoided wherever possible; **automated washer-disinfectors** are the preferred method.
- Instruments must be **visibly clean** prior to sterilisation.

Sterilisation

- Sterilisation must be carried out using validated **vacuum or non-vacuum steam sterilisers (autoclaves)**, appropriate to the instrument type.
- Practices must maintain documented records of **cycle parameters, routine testing, servicing, and maintenance**.

Packaging and Storage

- Sterilised instruments should be packaged where required and stored in **clean, dry, designated storage areas**.
- Stock rotation systems and, where applicable, expiry dates must be adhered to.

4. Environmental Cleaning and Zoning

- Dental surgeries should be organised into clearly defined **clean and contaminated zones** to reduce cross-contamination.[2]
- **High-touch surfaces** (e.g. door handles, light switches, keyboards, dental chairs) must be cleaned and disinfected between patients using approved products.
- **Dental unit waterlines (DUWLs)** must be maintained, flushed, and treated according to manufacturer instructions to control biofilm formation and microbial contamination.[6]

5. Waste and Sharps Management

- Clinical waste must be correctly **segregated, labelled, stored, and disposed of** in accordance with local policy and national waste regulations.
- Sharps must be disposed of **immediately after use** into approved sharps containers.
- **Safety-engineered sharps devices** should be used wherever reasonably practicable to reduce needlestick injury risk.[7]

6. Governance, Training, and Audit

- Every dental practice must appoint an **IPC Lead** responsible for oversight of infection control policies, training, and compliance.[4]
- All staff must receive **regular IPC training** appropriate to their role and responsibilities.
- Routine **audits and risk assessments** should be conducted to demonstrate compliance with HTM 01-05 and to support continuous improvement.

7. Patient Protection Measures

- Medical histories must be reviewed and updated at every visit to identify changes in health status or infection risk.
- The use of **rubber dam, high-volume suction, and effective ventilation** significantly reduces aerosol spread during dental procedures.[5]
- Patients should be provided with **clean protective eyewear and disposable bibs** where appropriate.

Summary

Infection prevention and control is a cornerstone of safe dental practice. By consistently applying standard precautions, maintaining effective decontamination systems, ensuring a clean clinical environment, and embedding strong governance and training frameworks, dental teams can minimise the risk of cross-infection and meet regulatory and professional expectations. A well-led IPC culture protects patients, staff, and the wider community and underpins public confidence in dental care.

References

1. Health and Social Care Act 2008 (Regulated Activities) Regulations 2014
2. Department of Health and Social Care. *HTM 01-05: Decontamination in Primary Care Dental Practices*
3. UK Health Security Agency. *National Infection Prevention and Control Manual*
4. Care Quality Commission (CQC). *Regulation 12: Safe Care and Treatment*
5. UK Health Security Agency & NHS England. *Guidance on Ventilation and Aerosol-Generating Procedures in Dentistry*
6. Public Health England. *Dental Unit Waterlines: Advice on Infection Control*
7. Health and Safety Executive. *Safe Use and Disposal of Sharps*

Communication, SBAR & Consent in Dental Practice

1. The Importance of Communication

Effective communication is fundamental to safe, ethical, and high-quality dental care. Clear communication:

- Protects patients from harm
- Builds trust, confidence, and rapport
- Reduces errors, misunderstandings, and complaints
- Ensures compliance with the **GDC Standards for the Dental Team**[8]

Dental professionals communicate not only with patients, but also with colleagues and external services, including **999 emergency services, general dental practitioners (GDPs), hospitals, and other healthcare providers.**

2. Communicating with Patients

Clear, Simple, and Accessible Communication

- Avoid clinical jargon; explain procedures in plain, understandable language
- Present information in manageable steps
- Check understanding using open-ended questions (e.g. "Can you tell me what you understand about the treatment?")

Patient-Centred Approach

- Listen actively and acknowledge patient concerns
- Adapt communication for patients with anxiety, learning disabilities, sensory impairment, or language barriers
- Use interpreters or communication aids where required
- Communication is a **two-way process**, not a one-sided explanation[8]

3. SBAR: A Structured Communication Tool

SBAR is a nationally recognised tool for the clear and concise transfer of clinical information, particularly in urgent or high-risk situations.[9]

Letter	Meaning	Purpose
S	Situation	What is happening now
B	Background	Relevant history or context
A	Assessment	What you think the problem is
R	Recommendation	What you need to happen next

Example: Dental Medical Emergency

- **S**: "This is a dental practice. I have a patient with suspected anaphylaxis."
- **B**: "They received local anaesthetic and developed wheeze and hypotension."
- **A**: "They are conscious but struggling to breathe."
- **R**: "We need an emergency ambulance urgently."

SBAR is particularly useful for:

- 999 emergency calls
- Handover to paramedics
- Escalating concerns within the dental team

4. Understanding Consent

Consent is a patient's agreement to treatment. For consent to be valid, it must be:

- **Voluntary**
- **Informed**
- **Given by a person with capacity**

These principles are set out in **GDC standards** and UK law.[810]

Types of Consent

- **Implied**: e.g. patient opens their mouth for examination
- **Verbal**: routine procedures
- **Written**: complex, invasive, or high-risk treatments

5. What Makes Consent Valid?

1. Capacity

Under the **Mental Capacity Act 2005**, a patient has capacity if they can:[10]

- Understand relevant information
- Retain that information
- Weigh it to make a decision
- Communicate their choice

Adults are presumed to have capacity unless proven otherwise.

2. Information

Patients must be informed about:

- The nature of the procedure
- Benefits and **material risks**
- Reasonable alternatives, including no treatment
- Costs, where relevant

3. Voluntariness

- Consent must be free from pressure or coercion
- Patients may withdraw consent at any time

Consent is an **ongoing process**, not a one-off signature.

6. Special Consent Situations

Children and Young People

- Assess **Gillick competence**
- If not competent, obtain consent from someone with **parental responsibility**[11]

Medical Emergencies

- If a patient lacks capacity and delay would risk serious harm or death, treatment may proceed in the patient's **best interests**
- The rationale must be clearly documented[10]

7. Documentation

Accurate and contemporaneous records must include:

- Information provided to the patient
- Questions asked and answers given
- Type of consent obtained
- Any refusal or withdrawal of consent

Good documentation protects both patients and the dental team.[8]

8. DNACPR (Do Not Attempt Cardiopulmonary Resuscitation) in Dental Practice

- A DNACPR is a **formal clinical decision** indicating that CPR should not be attempted in the event of cardiac arrest
- It applies **only to CPR**; all other appropriate care (e.g. oxygen, airway support, pain relief, comfort measures) must continue[12]

Respecting a DNACPR:

- Upholds patient autonomy and wishes
- Preserves dignity and comfort
- Prevents inappropriate or harmful interventions

Dental teams should:

- Be aware of existing DNACPR decisions when relevant
- Verify documentation where possible
- Follow national guidance if uncertainty exists[12]

9. Primary Survey: DRABCDE

The **DRABCDE** approach provides a rapid, systematic assessment to identify and manage **life-threatening conditions** and aligns with Resuscitation Council UK guidance.[13]

D – Danger

- Ensure the scene is safe
- Protect yourself, the patient, and others

R – Response

- Speak to the patient; gently shake shoulders
- If unresponsive, shout for help immediately

A – Airway

- Check airway is open and clear
- Remove visible obstructions and open the airway
- Airway compromise is **immediately life-threatening**

B – Breathing

- Look, listen, and feel for normal breathing
- Assess rate, depth, and effort
- Administer high-flow oxygen if available
- If breathing is absent or abnormal, **start CPR**

C – Circulation

- Check for signs of circulation and shock

- Control catastrophic bleeding immediately

D – Disability

- Assess consciousness using **AVPU**
- Check blood glucose if indicated
- Look for signs of seizure or stroke

E – Exposure

- Look for injuries, rashes, swelling, or medical alert jewellery
- Maintain patient warmth and dignity

References

8. General Dental Council. *Standards for the Dental Team*
9. NHS England. *SBAR Communication Tool Guidance*
10. Mental Capacity Act 2005 & Code of Practice
11. Department of Health. *Consent to Treatment of Children and Young People*
12. Resuscitation Council UK. *Decisions Relating to Cardiopulmonary Resuscitation*
13. Resuscitation Council UK. *Medical Emergencies and Resuscitation Standards for Clinical Practice*

Chain of Survival – Adult Cardiac Arrest

Chain of Survival

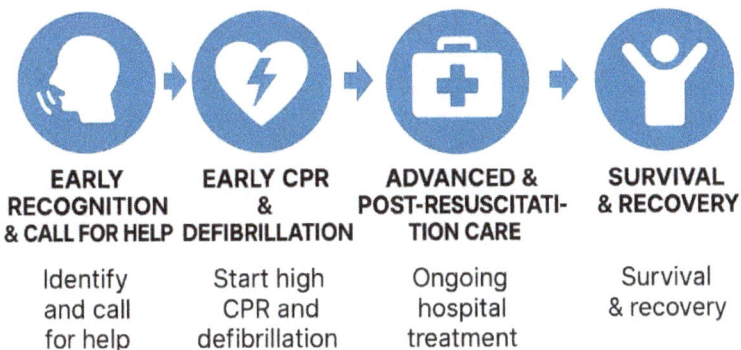

EARLY RECOGNITION & CALL FOR HELP	EARLY CPR & DEFIBRILLATION	ADVANCED & POST-RESUSCITATION CARE	SURVIVAL & RECOVERY
Identify and call for help	Start high CPR and defibrillation	Ongoing hospital treatment	Survival & recovery

The **Chain of Survival** describes the critical, time-sensitive actions required to maximise survival following adult cardiac arrest. Each link is equally important, and a delay at any stage reduces the chance of survival.[14]

1. Early Recognition and Call for Help

Prompt recognition of cardiac arrest and immediate activation of emergency services is the first and most crucial link.

- Check for **responsiveness**
- Open the airway and check for **normal breathing**
  - Occasional gasps or **agonal breathing are not normal breathing**
- If the patient is **unresponsive and not breathing normally**:
  - **Call 999 or 112 immediately**
  - **Send for the AED**

When calling emergency services, clearly state:

"Unresponsive adult, not breathing normally – suspected cardiac arrest."

Key point: Early recognition and early activation of emergency response is the single most important determinant of survival.[14]

2. Early CPR and Defibrillation

High-quality cardiopulmonary resuscitation (CPR) maintains vital organ perfusion and increases the likelihood that defibrillation will be successful.

Cardiopulmonary Resuscitation (CPR)

- Start CPR **immediately**
- Compression rate: **100–120 per minute**
- Compression depth: **5–6 cm**
- Allow **full chest recoil**
- Minimise interruptions
- Compression-to-ventilation ratio: **30 compressions: 2 breaths** (if trained and willing)
- If rescue breaths cannot be given safely, provide **compression-only CPR**

Defibrillation

- Apply the **AED as soon as it becomes available**
- Follow the AED voice and visual prompts
- Ensure **no one is touching the patient** during rhythm analysis
- Deliver a shock if advised
- **Resume CPR immediately** after the shock (do not reassess pulse or breathing)

Key point: CPR buys time by maintaining circulation; early defibrillation is the definitive treatment for shockable rhythms.[15]

3. Advanced Life Support and Post-Resuscitation Care

Once emergency services arrive, advanced care aims to stabilise the patient and address the cause of arrest.

This may include:

- Advanced airway management
- Oxygenation and ventilation
- Intravenous or intraosseous access
- Drug therapy
- Identification and treatment of **reversible causes** (e.g. hypoxia, hypovolaemia, thrombosis)

Role of the Dental Team

- Continue CPR until relieved by advanced providers
- Assist emergency services as requested
- Provide a clear, structured handover (e.g. SBAR)
- Preserve dignity and support staff and bystanders

4. Survival and Recovery

Survival from cardiac arrest extends beyond return of spontaneous circulation (ROSC) and includes long-term outcomes.

This stage focuses on:

- Ongoing hospital and critical care
- Neurological protection and monitoring
- Physical and psychological rehabilitation
- Follow-up and secondary prevention
- Team debrief and learning following the event

Key point: Successful resuscitation is measured not only by ROSC, but by meaningful survival and quality of recovery.[16]

Summary Table: Chain of Survival

Stage	Clinical Action
Early Recognition & Call for Help	Identify arrest, call 999/112
Early CPR & Defibrillation	High-quality CPR, rapid AED use
Advanced & Post-Resuscitation Care	ALS and hospital management
Survival & Recovery	Rehabilitation and long-term outcomes

Key Messages for Dental Practice

- **Unresponsive + not breathing normally = cardiac arrest**
- Call for help **first and fast**
- CPR and AED use must **never be delayed**
- Every dental practice must **train, rehearse, and audit** the Chain of Survival regularly[17]

References

14. Resuscitation Council UK. *Adult Basic Life Support Guidelines*
15. Resuscitation Council UK. *Defibrillation and Automated External Defibrillators*
16. Resuscitation Council UK. *Post-Resuscitation Care Guidelines*
17. Care Quality Commission. *Medical Emergencies in Primary Care*

Calling for Help and Assessing Vital Signs

1. Calling for Help

Early and effective communication with emergency services is critical during medical emergencies.

When calling **999 or 112** (or **2222 within NHS hospitals**), provide the following information clearly and calmly:

- **Your exact location**
  - Include practice name, full address, postcode, floor/room number if applicable
- **The type of help required**
  - For example: "Adult cardiac arrest", "Suspected anaphylaxis", "Unconscious patient"
- **Number of patients and casualties**
- **Patient details**
  - Age and sex (name if known)
- **Clear description of the situation**
  - Level of consciousness
  - Breathing status
  - Any immediate treatment already being provided

Do **not** end the call until instructed to do so by the emergency call handler.[18]

2. Assessing Vital Signs

Assessment of vital signs should be performed as part of a **systematic clinical assessment**, such as **DRABCDE**, and repeated regularly to detect deterioration.[19]

Airway

- Ensure the airway is **open and patent**
- Look for visible obstruction (e.g. foreign body, vomit, swelling)
- Listen for abnormal sounds such as stridor or gurgling

- If compromised, **airway management takes immediate priority**

Breathing

- Assess **rate, depth, rhythm, and effort**
- Normal adult respiratory rate: **12–20 breaths per minute**
- Measure oxygen saturation using pulse oximetry where available:
  - **Target SpO$_2$: 94–98%** in most adults
  - **Target SpO$_2$: 88–92%** in patients at risk of hypercapnic respiratory failure (e.g. COPD), if known[20]
- Look for signs of respiratory distress (cyanosis, accessory muscle use)

Circulation

Assess perfusion and cardiovascular status:

- **Pulse**
  - Check **carotid** pulse in unresponsive adults
  - Radial or brachial pulse may be used in conscious patients
  - Note rate, rhythm, and strength
- **Blood pressure**
  - Normal adult BP is approximately **120/80 mmHg**
  - Interpret in context of symptoms and baseline
- **Capillary refill time**
  - Normal: **≤2 seconds** (in adults, measured centrally if shocked)
- Look for signs of shock: pallor, sweating, tachycardia, hypotension[21]

Temperature

- Normal adult body temperature: **36.0–37.5°C**
- **Hypothermia**
  - Mild: **32–35°C**

- o Moderate: **28–32°C**
- o Severe: **<28°C**
- **Hyperthermia**
  - o **Heat exhaustion**: raised temperature with preserved consciousness
  - o **Heat stroke: core temperature ≥40°C with altered mental status**
    → This is a **medical emergency**[22]

Key Clinical Points for Practice

- Always **call for help early** if concerned
- Vital signs must be interpreted **together**, not in isolation
- Abnormal findings require **prompt escalation and reassessment**
- Repeated observations help identify **deterioration**

References (continuing numbering)

18. NHS England. *Emergency Call Handling and Communication Guidance*
19. Resuscitation Council UK. *Primary Survey and Assessment of the Acutely Ill Adult*
20. British Thoracic Society. *Guideline for Oxygen Use in Adults in Healthcare and Emergency Settings*
21. NICE. *Acutely Ill Adults in Hospital: Recognition and Response to Deterioration*
22. UK Health Security Agency. *Heat Illness and Hyperthermia Guidance*

Temperature

Digital Thermometer—This is the most accurate thermometer. It can take the temperature orally, in the armpit, or rectally.

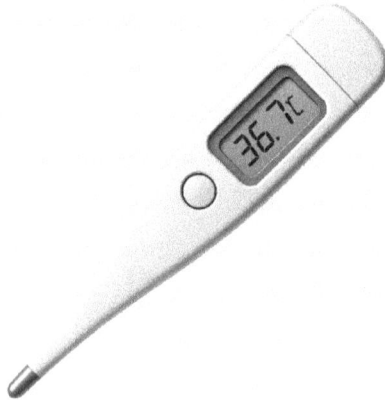

Tympanic Thermometer: is a thermometer that measures the temperature inside the patient's ears by measuring the infrared heat inside the ear.

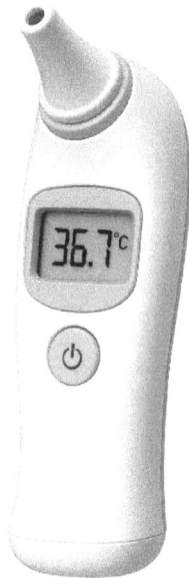

Temporal Thermometer-forehead thermometer. They are not as dependable as digital thermometers. They are placed or pointed at the forehead. They measure the infrared heat generated by the forehead.

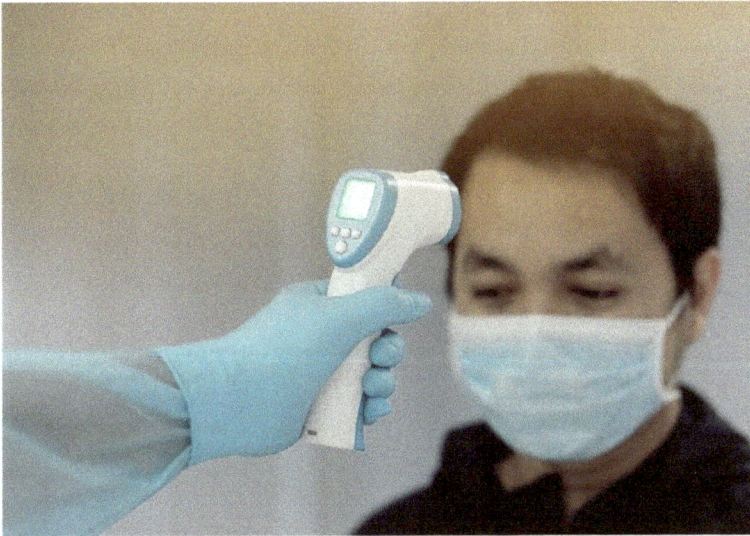

Pulse

The pulse is the palpable pressure wave produced by the contraction of the heart and the subsequent flow of blood through the arteries. It is used to assess **heart rate**, usually measured in beats per minute (bpm), and to evaluate the **rhythm, strength, and regularity** of cardiac activity.

Pulse Locations (Adult)

Peripheral and central pulse assessment is an essential component of clinical evaluation, particularly during medical emergencies. Pulse sites should be selected based on the patient's age, level of responsiveness, and clinical condition.[23]

Common Pulse Sites

Carotid Pulse (Central)

- Located on **either side of the neck**, in the groove between the trachea and the sternocleidomastoid muscle
- **Use one side only** to avoid compromising cerebral blood flow
- Primary site for pulse assessment in **unresponsive adults**[23]

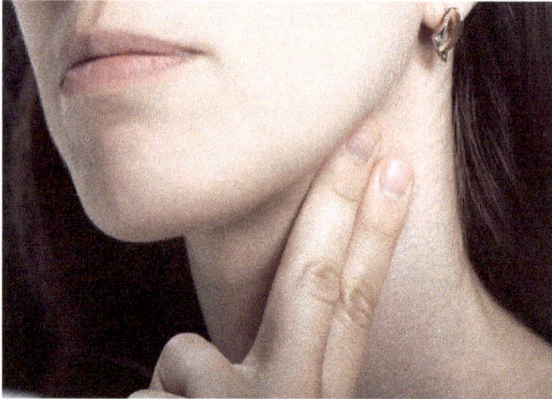

Brachial Pulse (Peripheral)

- Located on the **medial aspect of the upper arm**, between the biceps and triceps muscles
- More commonly used in **infants and children**, but may be used in adults when other pulses are difficult to palpate[24]

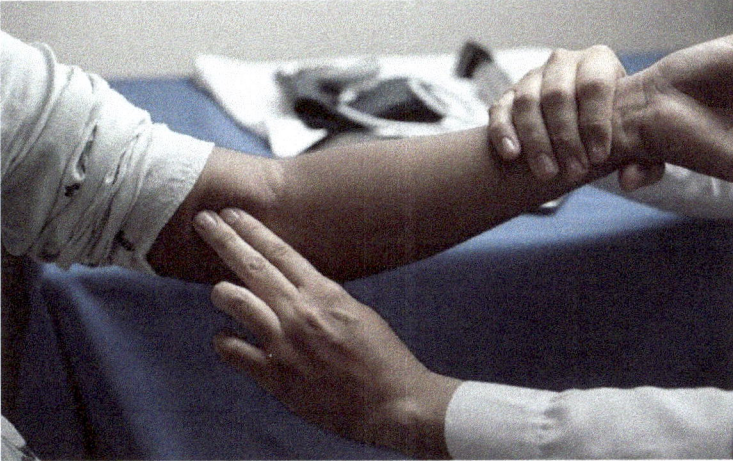

Femoral Pulse (Central)

- Located in the **upper thigh, just below the inguinal ligament**, midway between the anterior superior iliac spine and the pubic symphysis
- Useful in **shock, cardiac arrest, or low-flow states**[23]

Radial Pulse (Peripheral)

- Located on the **thumb side of the wrist**, between the radial bone and the flexor tendons
- Commonly used in **conscious adults** to assess rate and rhythm

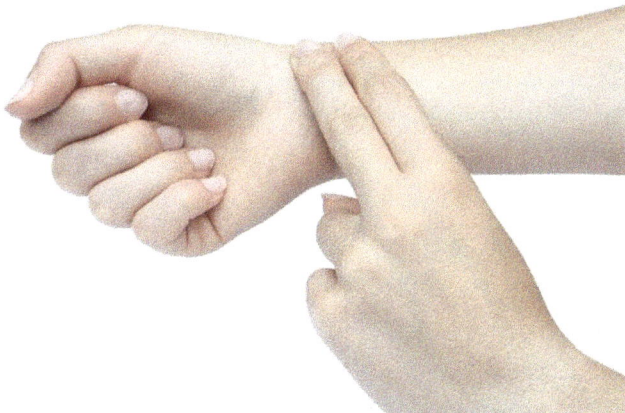

- Located behind the knee in the popliteal fossa
- Often difficult to palpate and requires the knee to ᵇ slightly flexed

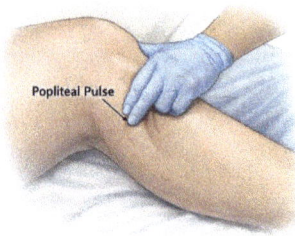

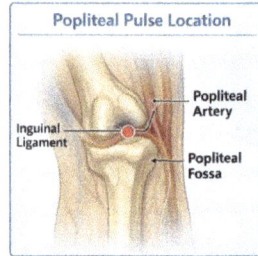

Popliteal Pulse Location

Popliteal Pulse

Inguinal Ligament

Popliteal Artery

Popliteal Fossa

Posterior Tibial Pulse (Peripheral)

- Located **behind and slightly below the medial malleolus** (inner ankle bone)
- Useful for assessing peripheral circulation in the lower limb

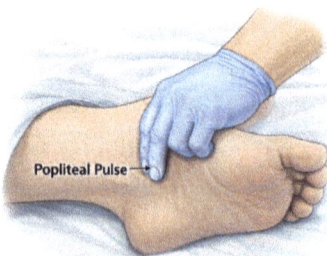

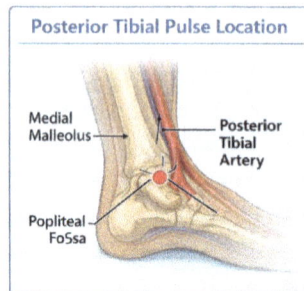

Posterior Tibial Pulse (Peripheral)

- Located behind and slightly below the medial malleolus (inner ankle bone)
- Useful for assessing peripheral circulation in the lower limb

Posterior Tibial Pulse Location

Popliteal Pulse

Medial Malleolus

Posterior Tibial Artery

Popliteal Fossa

Dorsalis Pedis Pulse (Peripheral)

- Located on the **dorsum (top) of the foot**, lateral to the extensor hallucis longus tendon

- May be absent in some healthy individuals and should be compared bilaterally[25]

Dorsalis Pedis Pulse (Peripheral)

- Located on the dorsum (top) of the foot, lateral to the extensor hallucis longus tendon
- May be absent in some healthy individuals and should be compared bilaterally[25]

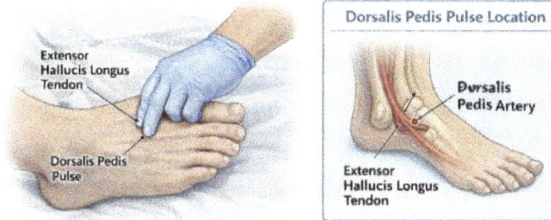

Dorsalis Pedis Pulse Location

Key Clinical Points

- In **unresponsive adults**, assess **carotid or femoral pulses**
- In **conscious patients**, radial pulse is usually sufficient
- Always assess **rate, rhythm, and strength** of the pulse
- Absence of a peripheral pulse does not always indicate cardiac arrest—assess alongside breathing and responsiveness

References

23. Resuscitation Council UK. *Adult Basic Life Support Guidelines*
24. Royal College of Paediatrics and Child Health. *Clinical Assessment of the Child*
25. NICE. *Peripheral Arterial Disease: Diagnosis and Management*

Pulse Oximeter

A pulse oximeter is a small, non-invasive device that clips onto a fingertip and uses light to measure oxygen saturation (SpO_2) and pulse rate.

It has no absolute contraindications, but readings may be unreliable with:

- Poor peripheral perfusion
- Movement or tremors
- Nail varnish or artificial nails
- Carbon monoxide exposure
- Severe anaemia
- Skin pigmentation or strong ambient light
- Incorrect placement or damaged sensors

It should support clinical assessment, not replace it.

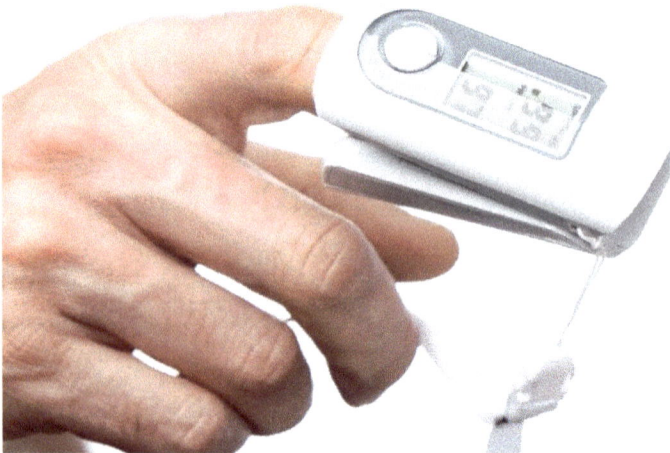

Blood Pressure Values (Adults)

Blood pressure (BP) is recorded as **systolic pressure over diastolic pressure** and is measured in millimetres of mercury (mmHg). Values should always be interpreted in the context of the patient's symptoms, clinical condition, and baseline readings.

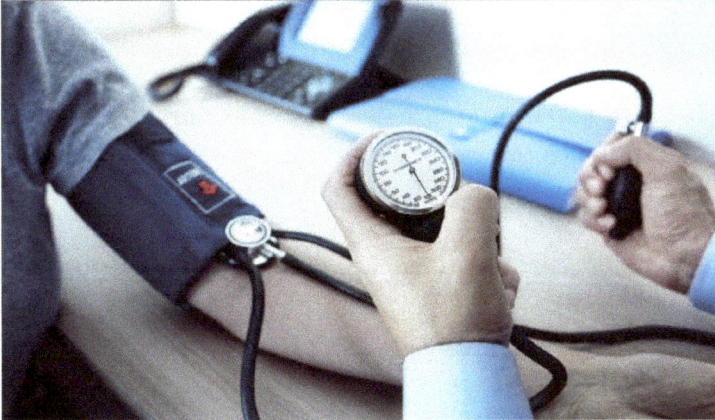

Normal Blood Pressure

- **Systolic: <120 mmHg**
- **Diastolic: <80 mmHg**

This range is associated with the lowest risk of cardiovascular disease in adults.[26]

Elevated Blood Pressure (High-Normal)

- **Systolic: 120–129 mmHg**
- **Diastolic: <80 mmHg**

Patients in this range are not classified as hypertensive but may require monitoring and lifestyle advice.[26]

Hypertension

Hypertension is diagnosed when blood pressure is **persistently elevated**:

- **Systolic: ≥140 mmHg**
- **Diastolic: ≥90 mmHg**

Diagnosis should be confirmed using repeated clinic readings, ambulatory blood pressure monitoring (ABPM), or home blood pressure monitoring (HBPM).[27]

Hypotension

- **Systolic: ≤90 mmHg**
- Often associated with symptoms such as dizziness, syncope, confusion, or signs of shock

Hypotension is clinically significant **when accompanied by symptoms or evidence of poor perfusion**, rather than by numerical value alone.[28]

Key Clinical Points for Practice

- Blood pressure should be interpreted alongside **pulse, respiratory rate, oxygen saturation, and level of consciousness**
- Sudden changes from a patient's normal baseline may indicate **acute illness or deterioration**
- In dental practice, **symptomatic hypotension or severe hypertension requires escalation and possible emergency referral**

References

26. NICE. *Hypertension in Adults: Diagnosis and Management (NG136)*
27. British & Irish Hypertension Society. *Guidelines for Blood Pressure Measurement and Classification*
28. Resuscitation Council UK. *Recognition and Management of the Acutely Ill Adult*

ASTHMA

Asthma is a long-term condition where inflamed, narrowed airways cause wheezing, coughing, and breathlessness.

Treatment starts with inhaled bronchodilators; if these are ineffective, intravenous medicines may be used to reduce bronchospasm and inflammation.

A reliever inhaler (e.g., salbutamol) opens the airways within minutes and is used only when symptoms occur, not routinely.

RELIEVER INHALER

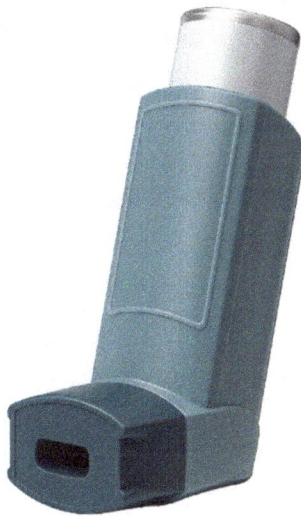

PREVENTER INHALER

A **preventer inhaler** is an asthma inhaler containing **inhaled corticosteroids** that is used **daily** to reduce airway inflammation and prevent asthma symptoms and attacks.

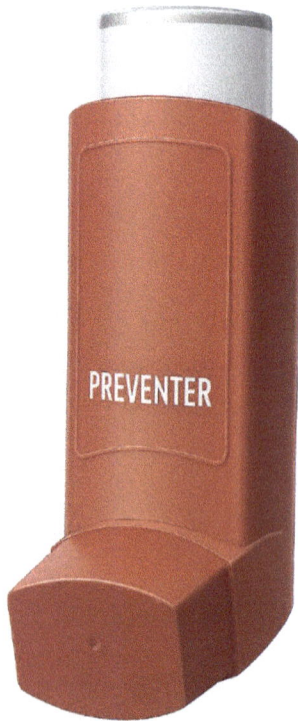

Salbutamol is a **beta₂ stimulant bronchodilator** that opens the airways by relaxing the muscles in the medium and small bronchi during spasm.

Salbutamol Overview

Feature	Summary
Drug type	Beta$_2$ stimulant bronchodilator
Action	Relaxes airway muscles and opens narrowed bronchi
Delivery	Often via oxygen-driven nebuliser
Onset	5–6 minutes
Peak effect	15–20 minutes
Duration	4–6 hours

PRESENTATION

Salbutamol nebulizer solution 5mg/2.5 ml

INDICATIONS

Salbutamol is used for acute asthma attacks in cases where regular inhaler therapy has not been effective in relieving the symptoms. It is also used in cases of expiratory wheezing due to allergy; anaphylaxis, smoke inhalation, or other lower airway causes or worsening chronic obstructive pulmonary disease.

Respiratory distress.

CONTRA-INDICATIONS

None in emergencies. Those with angioedema or patients with sensitivity to salbutamol. Use with caution when administering the medication to a patient who is a breastfeeding mother or patients with cardiovascular disorders or cardiac arrhythmias.

CAUTIONS

Salbutamol should be used with care in the following patients:

Hypertensive patients, angina, patients with overactive thyroid, and pregnant women in the late stages of pregnancy because the medication can lead to the relaxation of the uterus. Taking salbutamol can also lead to severe hypertension in patients on beta blockers- drugs that prevent the stimulation of adrenergic receptors responsible for increased cardiac action, used to control heart rhythm, angina attack, and high blood pressure. In patients with COPD, nebulization should be reduced to no more than 6 minutes.

SIDE EFFECTS

Tremor (shaking), Tachycardia (fast heartbeat), palpitations, headache, feeling of tension, muscle cramps, rash, and peripheral vasodilation.

DOSAGE AND ADMINISTRATION

Adult-5 mg/2.5ml nebulised 5-6 minutes. Give medication every 5 minutes until the patient recovers or the emergency services arrive.

Salbutamol & Related Medicines

1. Salbutamol Aerosol Inhaler (100 micrograms per puff)

Used with a **spacer** for fast relief of bronchospasm.

Aerosol Inhaler Doses

Medication	Age Group	Route	Dose	Repeat
Salbutamol inhaler	Children under 3 years	Inhaled via spacer	2–10 puffs	Every 10–20 minutes if needed
Salbutamol inhaler	Adults	Inhaled via spacer	2–10 puffs	Every 10–20 minutes if needed

2. Salbutamol Nebuliser Solution (1 mg/mL or 2 mg/mL)

Delivered via **oxygen-driven nebuliser** for moderate–severe symptoms.

Nebuliser Doses

Medication	Age Group	Route	Dose	Repeat
Salbutamol nebuliser	Children under 4 years	Oxygen-driven nebuliser	2.5 mg	Every 20–30 minutes if needed
Salbutamol nebuliser	Children 5–11 years	Nebuliser	2.5–5 mg	Every 20–30 minutes if needed
Salbutamol nebuliser	Children 12–17 years	Nebuliser	5 mg	Every 20–30 minutes if needed
Salbutamol nebuliser	Adults	Nebuliser	5 mg	Every 20–30 minutes if needed

3. Terbutaline Sulphate (2.5 mg/mL)

Alternative bronchodilator when salbutamol is unsuitable or ineffective.

Nebuliser Doses

Medication	Age Group	Route	Dose	Repeat
Terbutaline nebuliser	Under 4 years	Nebulised (oxygen-driven preferred)	5 mg	Every 20–30 minutes if needed

Medication	Age Group	Route	Dose	Repeat
Terbutaline nebuliser	5–11 years	Nebulised (oxygen-driven preferred)	5–10 mg	Every 20–30 minutes if needed
Terbutaline nebuliser	12–17 years	Nebulised (oxygen-driven preferred)	10 mg	Every 20–30 minutes if needed
Terbutaline nebuliser	Adults	Nebulised (oxygen-driven preferred)	10 mg	Every 20–30 minutes if needed

4. Prednisolone (tablets or soluble tablets)

Used alongside bronchodilators to reduce airway inflammation.

Prednisolone Doses

Medication	Age Group	Route	Dose	Duration
Prednisolone	Children under 11 years	Oral	1–2 mg/kg (max 40 mg)	Once daily for up to 3 days
If already on steroids	Children under 11 years	Oral	2 mg/kg (max 60 mg)	Once daily
Prednisolone	Children 12–17 years	Oral	40–50 mg	Once daily for ≥5 days
Prednisolone	Adults	Oral	40–50 mg	Once daily for ≥5 days

5. Hydrocortisone (sodium succinate)

Used when oral steroids are not possible.

Hydrocortisone Doses

Medication	Age Group	Route	Dose	Repeat
Hydrocortisone	Children under 17 years	IV	4 mg/kg (max 100 mg)	Every 6 hours until switched to oral steroids
Hydrocortisone	Child ≤1 year	IV	25 mg	As above
Hydrocortisone	Child 2–4 years	IV	50 mg	As above
Hydrocortisone	Child 5–17 years	IV	100 mg	As above
Hydrocortisone	Adults	IV	100 mg	Every 6 hours until switched to oral steroids

6. Ipratropium Bromide (Atrovent)

Added in moderate–severe asthma to improve bronchodilation.

Ipratropium Doses

Medication	Age Group	Route	Dose	Repeat
Ipratropium	Children under 11 years	Nebuliser (oxygen-driven preferred)	250 micrograms	Every 20–30 min for 2 hours, then every 4–6 hours if needed
Ipratropium	Children 12–17 years	Nebuliser (oxygen-driven preferred)	500 micrograms	Every 4–6 hours if needed

Medication	Age Group	Route	Dose	Repeat
Ipratropium	Adults	Nebuliser (oxygen-driven preferred)	500 micrograms	Every 6 hours

Seizures: Clinical Assessment & Emergency Management

1. What is a Seizure?

A seizure is a sudden burst of abnormal electrical activity in the brain, causing temporary changes in movement, behaviour, sensation, awareness, or consciousness.

Type depends on:

- The brain area involved
- Whether activity stays focal or becomes generalised

2. Generalised Tonic–Clonic Seizures (GTCS)

Most common seizure type.

Features

- **Tonic phase:** collapse, stiffening
- **Clonic phase:** rhythmic jerking
- Eyes open/rolled up, unresponsive
- Possible tongue biting, drooling, cyanosis, incontinence

Duration

- Usually **60–90 seconds**
- Followed by **post-ictal confusion, drowsiness, fatigue**

3. Epilepsy

A long-term condition causing recurrent, unprovoked seizures.

Common triggers

- Stroke or head injury
- Alcohol withdrawal

- Low blood sugar
- Drug toxicity
- CNS infection

4. Convulsive Status Epilepticus

A **medical emergency** defined as:

- A tonic–clonic seizure lasting **≥5 minutes**, OR
- Repeated seizures without recovery

Requires **immediate treatment**.

5. Focal Seizures

- Start in one brain area
- May stay focal or progress to GTCS
- Often preceded by an **aura**

Treat as GTCS if:

- Consciousness is impaired AND
- Seizure lasts **≥5 minutes**

Prolonged focal seizures (>60 min) risk permanent injury.

6. Phases of a Seizure

A. Prodrome (hours–days before)

Mood change, irritability, poor sleep, fatigue.

B. Aura (early ictal)

Déjà vu, unusual smells/tastes, visual changes, dizziness, tingling, nausea, sudden fear.

C. Ictal Phase

Active seizure: loss of awareness, jerking, abnormal sounds, lip smacking, sudden collapse or rigidity.

D. Post-Ictal Phase

Confusion, exhaustion, headache, nausea, temporary weakness, incontinence, emotional distress.

7. Assessment & Initial Management

Safety

- Protect from injury
- After seizure stops, place in **recovery position**

History

Witness account, duration, known epilepsy, triggers, alcohol/drugs, pregnancy, medications.

Airway

- Maintain airway
- OPA only if tolerated
- NPA unless facial trauma suspected

Breathing

- Check rate, effort, SpO_2
- Give **15 L/min oxygen** during GTCS
- Target SpO_2: **94–98%** (adults), **88–92%** (COPD)
- Assist ventilation if needed
- **Do not delay benzodiazepines** in ongoing convulsions

Circulation & Injuries

- Check pulse, glucose

- Look for head injury, tongue bite, incontinence, rash
- Consider pregnancy/eclampsia

8. When to Give Emergency Benzodiazepines

Give if:

- Seizure lasts ≥**5 minutes**, OR
- **≥3 seizures in 1 hour**, OR
- Ongoing seizure without recovery

9. Buccal Midazolam

- Pre-filled syringes: **2.5 mg, 5 mg, 7.5 mg, 10 mg**
- Give buccally (between gum and cheek)
- May repeat once after **5–10 minutes**

10. Rectal Diazepam – Quick Reference Table

Diazepam Rectal Solution (2 mg/mL or 4 mg/mL)

Age Group	Route	Dose	Repeat
Neonates	Rectal	1.25–2.5 mg	Once after 5–10 min
1 month–1 year	Rectal	5 mg	Once after 5–10 min
2–11 years	Rectal	5–10 mg	Once after 5–10 min
12–17 years	Rectal	10–20 mg	Once after 5–10 min
Adults	Rectal	10–20 mg	Once after 5–10 min
Elderly	Rectal	10 mg	Once after 5–10 min

11. Midazolam Oromucosal (Buccal) – Quick Reference Table

Age Group	Route	Dose	Repeat
Neonates	Buccal	300 micrograms/kg	Once after 5–10 min

Age Group	Route	Dose	Repeat
1–2 months	Buccal	300 micrograms/kg (max 2.5 mg)	Once after 5–10 min
3–11 months	Buccal	2.5 mg	Once after 5–10 min
1–4 years	Buccal	5 mg	Once after 5–10 min
5–9 years	Buccal	7.5 mg	Once after 5–10 min
≥10 years & adults	Buccal	10 mg	Once after 5–10 min

Clinical Safety Considerations

Cautions

Increased risk of respiratory depression or arrest in:

- children
- older adults
- chronically unwell patients
- those intoxicated with alcohol
- patients taking other sedatives

Contraindications

- None in life-threatening convulsive status epilepticus
- Use with caution where airway compromise is likely

Possible Side Effects

- confusion or amnesia
- hypotension
- reduced consciousness
- respiratory depression

A seizure lasting **five minutes or longer** is a medical emergency. Early administration of benzodiazepines and prompt escalation according to local protocols are essential.

Any seizure lasting **5 minutes or longer** should be treated as a **medical emergency**, with early benzodiazepine administration and escalation according to local protocols.

Patient Group Directions (PGDs) and Exemptions: Summary for Dental Practice

1. Patient Group Directions (Current Framework)

A Patient Group Direction (PGD) is a legally authorised document that allows named, trained, and registered healthcare professionals to supply or administer specified medicines to defined groups of patients without an individual prescription.

PGDs must be developed and approved through local clinical governance systems, usually involving a doctor, a pharmacist, and relevant stakeholders.

Before June 2024, dental hygienists and dental therapists could use PGDs to administer certain medicines within their scope of practice, provided appropriate governance was in place.

2. Amendments to the Human Medicines Regulations (from 26 June 2024)

The Human Medicines Regulations 2012 were amended to allow registered dental hygienists and dental therapists to **sell, supply, and administer specified medicines within their professional scope without a prescription, PSD, or PGD**.

This applies across the UK and is enabled through the **exemptions** listed in Schedule 17 of the Regulations.

Practical Effect

Dental hygienists and therapists may now supply or administer certain prescription-only and pharmacy medicines directly, without:

- a dentist's prescription
- a Patient Specific Direction (PSD)
- a Patient Group Direction (PGD)

3. Understanding Exemptions

Exemptions allow dental hygienists and therapists to supply or administer specified medicines relevant to their clinical practice, provided they are trained, competent, and working within scope.

Exemptions **do not** grant prescribing rights; they simply remove the need for a prescription or PGD for medicines listed in the exemption framework.

4. Examples of Medicines Covered by Exemptions

Under the current exemptions, dental hygienists and therapists may supply or administer:

- certain local anaesthetics
- high-strength fluoride preparations
- other medicines relevant to dental care and within their competence

They must ensure appropriate training, competence, and indemnity.

5. PGDs vs Exemptions

When PGDs Still Apply

PGDs remain relevant for:

- healthcare professionals not covered by exemptions
- medicines or clinical situations outside the exemption list
- wider community or acute care settings

Where an exemption applies, it should be used instead of a PGD.

What Has Changed

- **Before June 2024:** Dental hygienists and therapists relied on PGDs or PSDs for many prescription-only medicines.
- **After June 2024:** They may use exemptions to supply or administer specified medicines directly, removing the legal requirement for PGDs in those cases.

6. Professional Standards

Regulators such as the General Dental Council expect dental hygienists and dental therapists to:

- be trained and competent in the use of exemptions
- work strictly within their scope of practice
- maintain patient safety and professional accountability

Use of exemptions is optional; PGDs or PSDs may still be used where appropriate, provided all legal and professional requirements are met.

Key Points

- Dental hygienists and dental therapists may now supply or administer certain medicines without a PGD under the exemptions framework.
- They **cannot prescribe** medicines.
- They must be trained, competent, indemnified, and acting within scope.
- PGDs remain relevant for medicines not covered by exemptions.

POSITIONAL TREATMENT FOR SEIZURE-RECOVERY POSITION

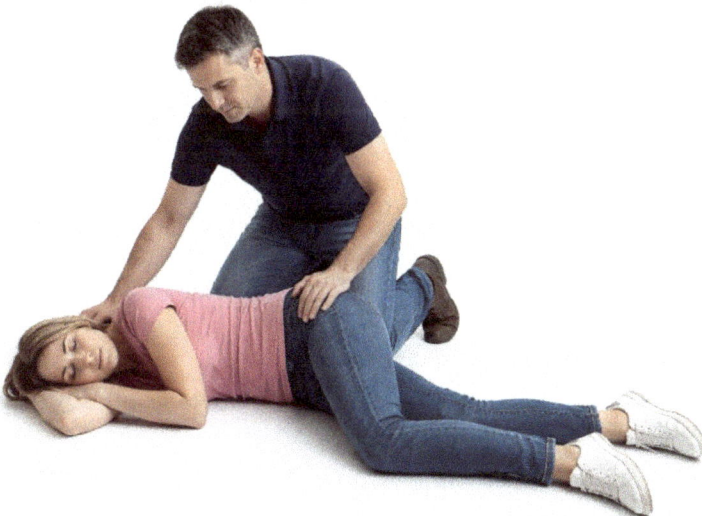

The **recovery position** is a **first-aid technique** used to keep a **breathing but unconscious** person safe while you wait for help.

What is the recovery position?

It is a **side-lying position** that:

- Keeps the **airway open**
- Allows fluids (vomit, saliva, blood) to **drain from the mouth**
- Reduces the risk of **airway obstruction or aspiration**

When is it used?

Use the recovery position if a person:

- Is **unconscious but breathing normally**
- Has had a **seizure** and is now in the post-ictal phase
- Has fainted
- Is unresponsive due to illness or injury (and spinal injury is not suspected)

Do not use if the person is not breathing normally — start CPR instead.

Why is it important?

The recovery position:

- Prevents the tongue from falling back and blocking the airway
- Reduces choking risk if the person vomits
- Allows continuous monitoring of breathing

Key features of the correct position

- Person lying **on their side**
- **Head tilted slightly back** to keep the airway open
- **Mouth facing downward** to allow drainage
- **Top leg bent** at the hip and knee to prevent rolling
- **Hand supporting the head**

Clinical and first-aid relevance

- Recommended by **NICE, Resuscitation Council UK, and JRCALC**
- Standard care following **tonic–clonic seizures** once convulsions stop
- Used in **pre-hospital, workplace, and community first-aid settings**

When to seek help

Call emergency services if:

- Breathing becomes abnormal
- Another seizure occurs
- The person does not regain consciousness as expected
- The seizure lasted **5 minutes or more**
- There are injuries or pregnancy concerns

Stroke & Transient Ischaemic Attack (TIA)

1. What Is a Stroke?

A stroke occurs when blood flow to part of the brain is interrupted, causing rapid brain injury.
Types:

- **Ischaemic stroke** – blockage of a cerebral blood vessel (most common)
- **Haemorrhagic stroke** – bleeding into or around the brain

Stroke is a time-critical medical emergency.

2. Who Can Have a Stroke?

Stroke can occur at any age. Risk increases with age, but children and young adults can also be affected. Early recognition and rapid hospital treatment improve outcomes.

3. Signs and Symptoms

Sudden onset of:

- Facial, arm, or leg weakness or numbness (usually one-sided)
- Slurred or unclear speech, difficulty understanding speech
- Visual loss or disturbance
- Loss of balance or coordination
- Severe headache (more common in haemorrhage)
- Nausea, vomiting, dizziness
- Confusion or reduced consciousness
- Seizure at onset
- Neck pain or stiffness (possible subarachnoid haemorrhage)

4. FAST Assessment (Recommended by NICE & RCUK)

A rapid screening tool for suspected stroke:

- **F – Face:** Facial droop or uneven smile
- **A – Arms:** Weakness or inability to lift one arm
- **S – Speech:** Slurred, confused, or absent speech
- **T – Time:** Call **999** immediately

5. Transient Ischaemic Attack (TIA)

A TIA is a brief interruption of cerebral blood flow causing stroke-like symptoms that fully resolve within 24 hours (usually minutes). A TIA is a **warning sign** with a high short-term risk of stroke. Symptoms mirror stroke and require **urgent medical assessment**.

6. Immediate Management (Pre-Hospital)

- Call **999/112** and state **"suspected stroke"**
- Note the **time symptoms started** or **last known well**

Airway & Breathing

- Monitor continuously

- If unconscious but breathing: **recovery position**
- If conscious: lie flat with head slightly elevated (unless hypotensive)

Do NOT

- Give food, drink, or medication
- Allow the person to walk
- Delay emergency services

7. Why Time Matters

- Brain cells die rapidly during a stroke
- Treatments such as **thrombolysis** and **thrombectomy** are highly time-dependent
- Early hospital arrival improves survival and long-term recovery

Key Points

- Stroke is a **medical emergency** at any age
- Use **FAST** for rapid recognition
- **TIA is urgent** and must not be dismissed
- Call **999/112** immediately
- Support airway, breathing, and safe positioning while awaiting help

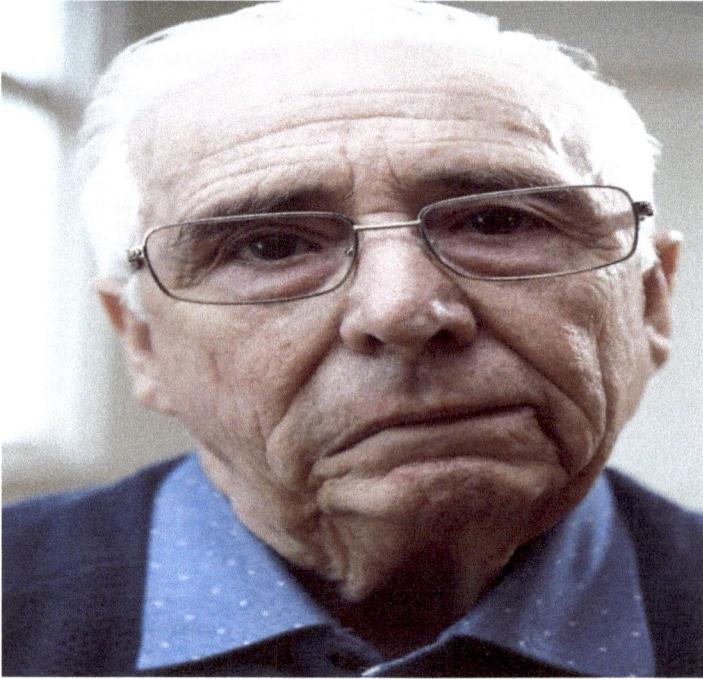

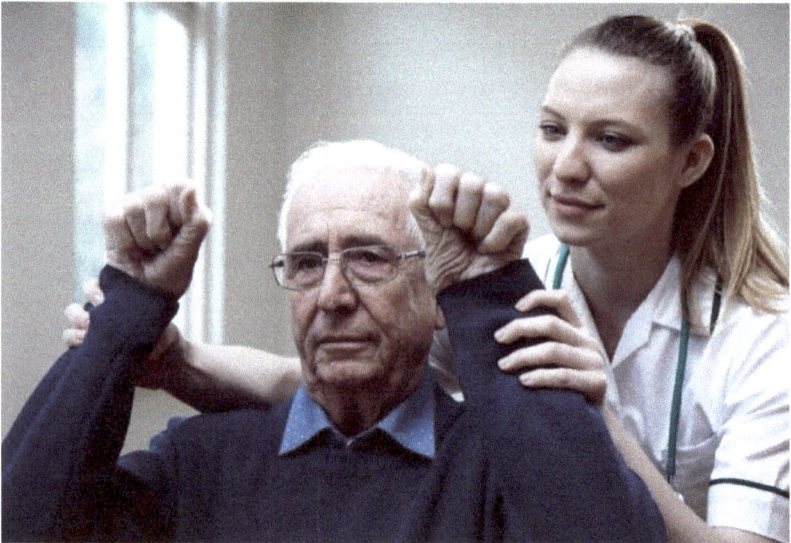

THE HEART: STRUCTURE, FUNCTION, AND CARDIAC EMERGENCIES

1. Structure of the Heart

The heart is a **muscular pump** responsible for circulating blood around the body. It has **four chambers**:

Upper chambers (Atria)

Right atrium- The **right atrium** is one of the **four chambers of the heart**, located in the **upper right side**. Its key role is to **receive deoxygenated blood** from the body and pass it to the **right ventricle**, which then pumps it to the lungs for oxygenation.-

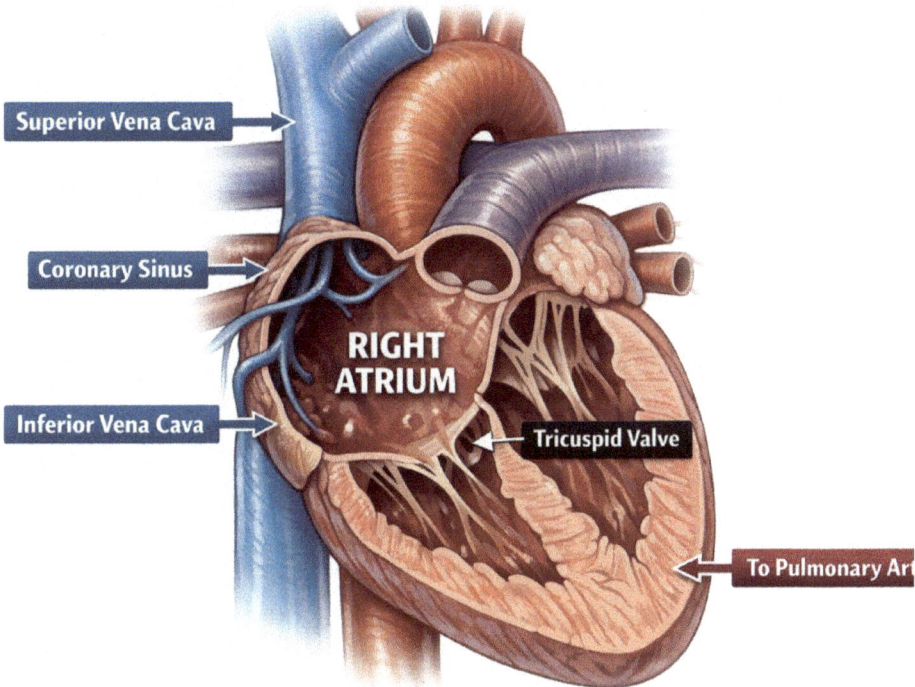

Left atrium-The **left atrium** is one of the four chambers of the heart. Its primary role is to **receive oxygen-rich blood from the lungs** through the **pulmonary veins** and then **pump it into the left ventricle**, which sends it out to the rest of the body. Key points about the left atrium:

- **Location:** Upper left side of the heart.
- **Function:** Acts as a holding chamber for blood returning from the lungs.
- **Connection:** Blood flows from the left atrium through the **mitral valve** into the left ventricle.

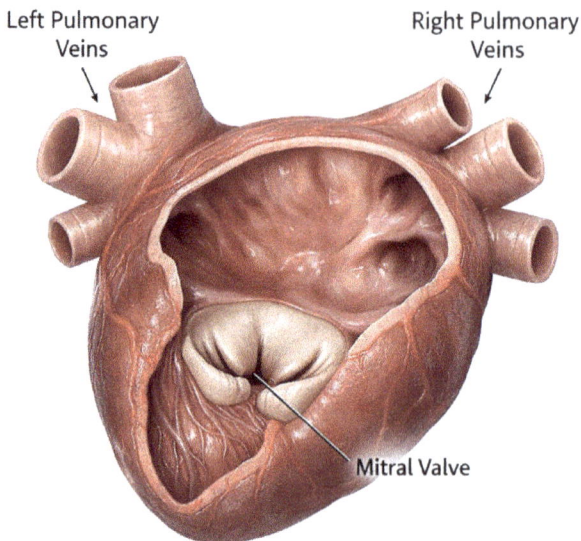

Left Pulmonary Veins

Right Pulmonary Veins

Mitral Valve

Left Atrium

Lower chambers (ventricles)

Right ventricle-The **right ventricle** is one of the four chambers of the heart.

In simple terms:

- It is the **lower right chamber** of the heart.

- Its job is to **pump deoxygenated (low oxygen) blood to the lungs**.

How it works:

1. Deoxygenated blood enters the **right atrium** from the body.
2. Blood flows from the right atrium into the **right ventricle**.
3. When the right ventricle contracts, it pumps blood through the **pulmonary valve** into the **pulmonary artery**.
4. The blood then travels to the **lungs**, where it picks up oxygen.

Key features:

- Has a **thinner muscular wall** than the left ventricle because it pumps blood at **lower pressure** (only to the lungs, not the whole body).
- Plays a vital role in **oxygenation of blood** and overall circulation.

Why it is important:

If the right ventricle fails, blood can back up in the body, causing symptoms such as **leg swelling, abdominal swelling, and breathlessness**.

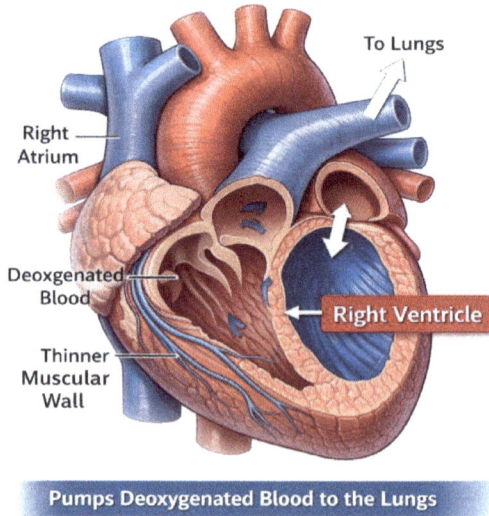

Right Atrium

To Lungs

Deoxgenated Blood

Right Ventricle

Thinner Muscular Wall

Pumps Deoxygenated Blood to the Lungs

Left ventricle-The **left ventricle** is one of the four chambers of the heart. Its key role is to **pump oxygen-rich blood around the body**.

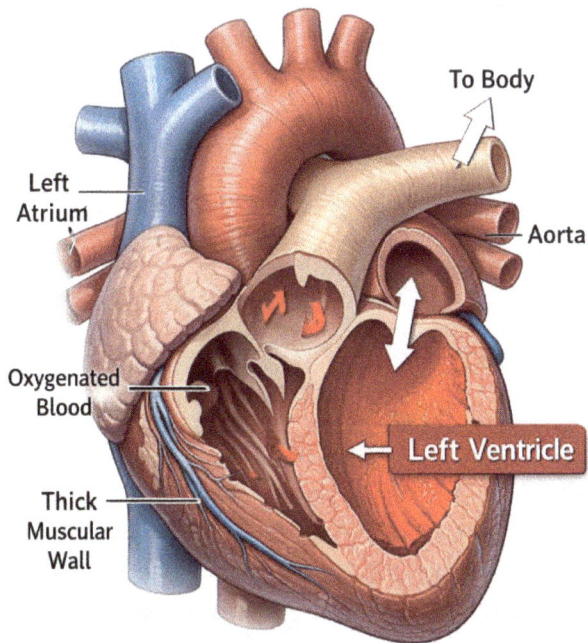

Left Atrium

To Body

Aorta

Oxygenated Blood

Left Ventricle

Thick Muscular Wall

Pumps Oxygen-Rich Blood to the Body

Key points:

- It receives oxygenated blood from the **left atrium**
- It pumps this blood into the **aorta**, the body's largest artery
- From the aorta, blood is delivered to all organs and tissues
- It has **thick muscular walls** because it must generate high pressure to circulate blood throughout the body

Why it is important:

The left ventricle is the heart's main pumping chamber. If it does not work correctly, organs may not receive enough oxygen, leading to conditions such as **heart failure** or **shock**.

2. Function of the Right and Left Sides of the Heart

Right Side of the Heart

- Receives **deoxygenated blood** from the body.
- Pumps blood to the **lungs** for oxygenation via the pulmonary circulation.

Left Side of the Heart

- Receives **oxygenated blood** from the lungs
- Pumps blood to the **rest of the body** via the systemic circulation

3. Blood Vessels

- **Arteries** – carry blood **away from the heart** (usually oxygenated)
- *Coronary arteries* supply the heart muscle itself
- **Veins** – return **deoxygenated blood** to the heart
- **Capillaries** – tiny vessels where **oxygen and nutrient exchange** occur.

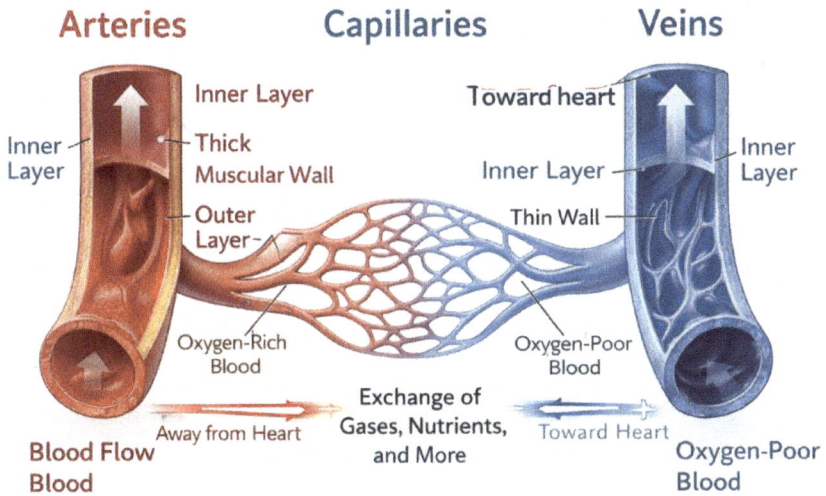

Arteries   Capillaries   Veins

Inner Layer

Inner Layer

Thick Muscular Wall

Toward heart

Inner Layer

Inner Layer

Outer Layer

Thin Wall

Oxygen-Rich Blood

Oxygen-Poor Blood

Away from Heart

Exchange of Gases, Nutrients, and More

Toward Heart

Blood Flow

Oxygen-Poor Blood

Blood

4. Heart Valves

Valves ensure **one-way blood flow** through the heart.

Right Side Valves

- **Tricuspid valve** – right atrium → right ventricle
- **Pulmonary valve** – right ventricle → lungs

Left Side Valves

- **Mitral (bicuspid) valve** – left atrium → left ventricle
- **Aortic valve** – left ventricle → aorta

5. Layers of the Heart

- **Pericardium** – protective outer sac
- **Myocardium** – muscular layer responsible for contraction
- **Endocardium** – smooth inner lining of chambers and valves

Septum

- Separates the left and right sides of the heart
- Prevents mixing of oxygenated and deoxygenated blood

6. How Oxygenated Blood Circulates

1. Right atrium receives deoxygenated blood
2. Right ventricle pumps blood to lungs
3. Left atrium receives oxygenated blood
4. Left ventricle pumps blood to the body

7. The Heart's Electrical (Conduction) System

The heart beats due to an internal electrical system:

- **Sinoatrial (SA) node** – natural pacemaker (60–100 bpm)
- **Atrioventricular (AV) node** – delays impulse to allow ventricular filling
- **Bundle of His** – transmits impulse to ventricles
- **Purkinje fibres** – coordinate ventricular contraction

Autonomic Control

- **Sympathetic system** – increases heart rate
- **Parasympathetic system** – slows heart rate

Cardiac Conduction System — Explained Simply and Clearly

The **cardiac conduction system** is the heart's **electrical wiring**. It controls **when and how the heart beats**, ensuring the chambers contract in the correct order to pump blood effectively.

1. Sinoatrial (SA) Node – *The natural pacemaker*

- Located in the **right atrium**
- Generates electrical impulses automatically
- Sets the normal heart rate (**60–100 bpm** in adults)

- Each impulse starts one heartbeat

→ This is why Normal Sinus Rhythm is called *sinus* rhythm.

2. Atrial Pathways

- Electrical impulse spreads across both atria
- Causes the **atria to contract**
- Pushes blood into the ventricles

→ This produces the **P wave** on the ECG.

3. Atrioventricular (AV) Node – *The delay point*

- Located between the atria and ventricles
- **Briefly delays** the electrical signal
- Allows ventricles time to fill with blood

→ The delay is vital for efficient cardiac output.

4. Bundle of His

- Conducts the impulse from the AV node into the ventricles
- Only normal electrical connection between atria and ventricles

5. Right and Left Bundle Branches

- Run down the interventricular septum
- Carry impulses to each ventricle
- Left branch splits into anterior and posterior fascicles

6. Purkinje Fibres

- Spread rapidly through ventricular muscle
- Cause **strong, coordinated ventricular contraction**

→ This produces the **QRS complex** on the ECG.

ECG Summary

ECG Component	Electrical Event
P wave	Atrial depolarisation
PR interval	AV node delay
QRS complex	Ventricular depolarisation
T wave	Ventricular repolarisation

Clinical importance (Resuscitation context)

- Disruption can cause **bradycardia, tachycardia, heart block, VF, or VT**
- Cardiac arrest rhythms occur when this system **fails or becomes chaotic**
- Defibrillation aims to **reset abnormal conduction**

8. Cardiac Rhythms

Normal Sinus Rhythm (NSR) is the **normal, healthy heart rhythm.**

What it means:

- The heartbeat starts from the **sinoatrial (SA) node**, the heart's natural pacemaker.
- Electrical impulses travel through the heart in an **organised and predictable way**.

Key features:

- **Regular rhythm**
- **Heart rate: 60–100 beats per minute (bpm)** in adults
- Each heartbeat has:
  - A **P wave** (atrial contraction)
  - Followed by a **QRS complex** (ventricular contraction)
  - Then a **T wave** (ventricular relaxation)

Why it is not shockable:

- Defibrillation is used for **chaotic or disorganised rhythms** (e.g. ventricular fibrillation).
- Normal Sinus Rhythm is **organised**, so a shock would **not help and could be harmful**.

Clinical significance (basic life support context):

- If a patient has NSR, the heart is **electrically and mechanically functioning**.
- Cardiac arrest rhythms are **not NSR**.

Normal Sinus Rhythm

- Regular rhythm, 60–100 bpm
- Not a shockable rhythm

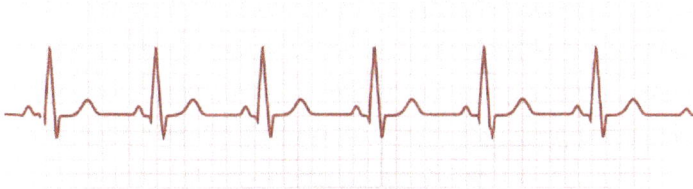

Normal Sinus Rhythm

Ventricular Fibrillation (VF)

Ventricular fibrillation (VF) is a **life-threatening cardiac arrest rhythm**.

What it is

Ventricular fibrillation occurs when the **ventricles quiver chaotically instead of contracting normally**. The heart's electrical activity becomes completely disorganised, so **no effective cardiac output** is produced.

What happens in the heart

- Electrical impulses fire **randomly and rapidly**
- Ventricles **do not pump blood**
- **Circulation stops immediately**
- The person becomes **unconscious within seconds** and will die without rapid treatment

ECG characteristics

- **Chaotic, irregular waveform**
- **No identifiable P waves, QRS complexes, or T waves**
- May appear **coarse** (large waves) or **fine** (small waves)

Why it is shockable:

- VF is caused by **disorganised electrical activity**
- **Defibrillation** delivers a controlled shock to:
  - Stop the chaotic activity
  - Allow the heart's natural pacemaker to restart a normal rhythm

Clinical importance (BLS / ALS context)

- VF is a **shockable cardiac arrest rhythm**
- Management includes:
  - **Immediate CPR**
  - **Early defibrillation**
  - Advanced life support and reversible cause management (4 Hs & 4 Ts)

Now generating a clear ECG illustration of **Ventricular Fibrillation**.

Ventricular Fibrillation

- Chaotic, disorganised electrical activity
- No effective pumping of blood

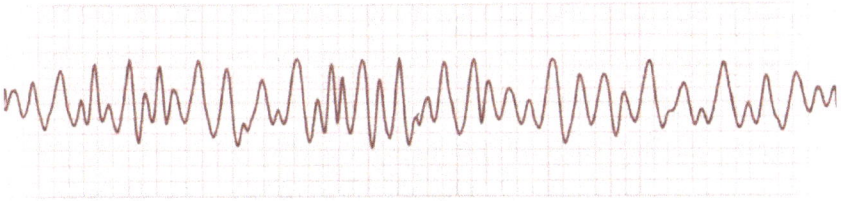

Ventricular Fibrillation

- Chaotic electrical activity
- **Shockable** rhythm

Pulseless Ventricular Tachycardia (VT)

Pulseless ventricular tachycardia (pVT) is a **life-threatening cardiac arrest rhythm** where the heart has electrical activity but **no effective cardiac output**.

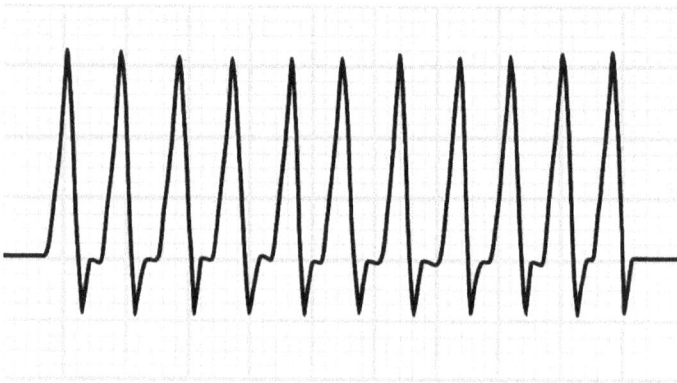

Pulseless Ventricular Tachycardia

What it is

- A **fast, abnormal rhythm** originating from the **ventricles**
- Ventricles contract **so rapidly and inefficiently** that they **cannot fill or pump blood**
- **No palpable pulse**, despite organised electrical activity

The patient is in **cardiac arrest**.

ECG features

- **Regular, wide-complex tachycardia**
- Rate usually **>150–250 bpm**
- **No visible P waves**
- QRS complexes are **wide and uniform** (monomorphic) or variable (polymorphic)

Why there is no pulse

- Extreme rate → **no ventricular filling time**
- Poor coordination → **ineffective contraction**
- Cardiac output falls to **zero**

Why it is shockable

- pVT is caused by **organised but dangerous electrical activity**
- **Defibrillation** can interrupt the rhythm
- Allows the heart's natural pacemaker to re-establish control
  pVT is a **shockable rhythm** (like VF)

Clinical presentation

- Unconscious
- Not breathing normally (or apnoeic)
- **No central pulse**
- Collapse may be sudden

Management

- **Immediate CPR**
- **Defibrillation ASAP**
- Adrenaline and amiodarone per ALS algorithm
- Identify and treat **reversible causes (4 Hs & 4 Ts)**

Difference from VT with a pulse

Feature	VT with pulse	Pulseless VT
Pulse	Present	**Absent**
Blood pressure	Low/unstable	**None**
Consciousness	May be reduced	**Unconscious**
Management	Cardioversion/antiarrhythmics	**CPR + defibrillation**

Asystolic rhythm (Asystole)

Asystole is a **cardiac arrest rhythm** in which there is **no electrical activity in the heart**. It is commonly referred to as **"flatline."** Because there is no electrical impulse, there is **no cardiac contraction and no cardiac output**, making it a **medical emergency with an extremely poor prognosis**.

Key characteristics

- **ECG appearance:** Near-flat line with no P waves, QRS complexes, or T waves
- **Heart activity:** None (no depolarisation)
- **Pulse:** Absent
- **Blood pressure:** Absent
- **Shockable rhythm:** No (defibrillation is not effective)

Common causes (Hs and Ts)

- **Hypoxia**
- **Severe acidosis**
- **Hypovolemia**
- **Electrolyte imbalance (especially potassium)**
- **Massive myocardial infarction**
- **Drug overdose**
- **Prolonged cardiac arrest**

Management

- Immediate **high-quality CPR**
- **Epinephrine** administration
- **Identify and treat reversible causes**
- Confirm rhythm is true asystole (check leads, gain, loose electrodes)

ECG illustration of asystole

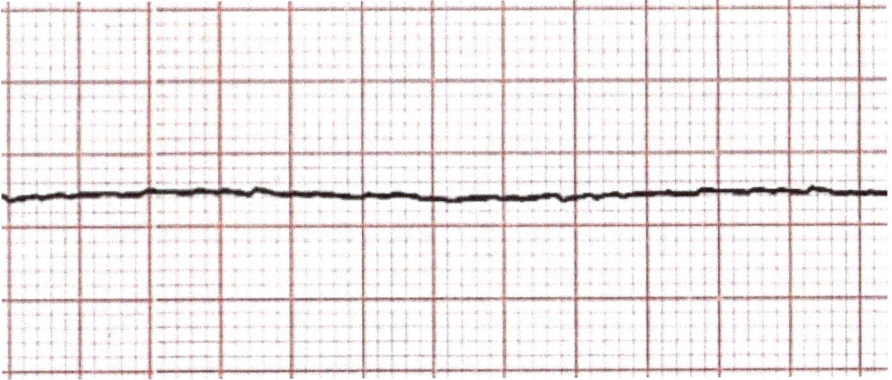

10. Acute Coronary Syndromes (ACS)

ACS describes conditions caused by **reduced blood flow to the heart muscle**:

- Stable angina
- Unstable angina
- Non-ST elevation myocardial infarction (NSTEMI)
- ST elevation myocardial infarction (STEMI)

11. Angina

Stable Angina

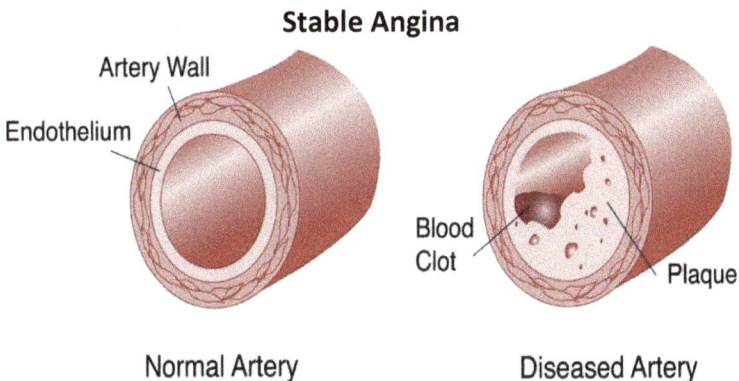

Artery Wall

Endothelium

Blood Clot

Plaque

Normal Artery

Diseased Artery

Stable angina is a type of **chest pain or discomfort** caused by **reduced blood flow to the heart muscle** (myocardial ischaemia), usually due to **coronary artery disease**.

What happens

- The coronary arteries are **narrowed by atherosclerosis**
- At rest, blood flow may be adequate
- During **exertion, stress, or cold**, the heart needs more oxygen
- The narrowed arteries **cannot meet this increased demand**
- This causes **temporary ischaemia → chest pain**

Key features (classic pattern)

- **Predictable**: occurs with the same level of exertion
- **Relieved by rest** or **glyceryl trinitrate (GTN)**
- Lasts **minutes (usually <10–15 minutes)**
- Does **not cause permanent heart damage**

Typical symptoms

- Central chest **tightness, pressure, or heaviness**
- Pain may **radiate** to the left the arm, neck, jaw, or back
- Associated:
  - Breathlessness
  - Sweating
  - Nausea
  - Fatigue

Common triggers

- Physical exertion
- Emotional stress
- Wintry weather
- Heavy meals

How it differs from unstable angina / MI

Feature	Stable Angina	Unstable Angina / MI
Pattern	Predictable	Unpredictable
Occurs at rest	No	Yes (often)

Feature	Stable Angina	Unstable Angina / MI
Relief	Rest / GTN	Often poor
Duration	Short	Prolonged
Myocardial damage	No	Possible / likely

Diagnosis (UK context)

- Clinical history is key
- ECG may be normal at rest
- Functional testing or CT coronary angiography per **NICE guidance**
- Troponin is **normal**

Management

Lifestyle:

- Smoking cessation
- Exercise
- Diet and weight management

Medication:

- **GTN** for symptom relief
- **Beta-blockers** or **calcium channel blockers**
- **Antiplatelets** (e.g. aspirin)
- **Statins**

Revascularisation if symptoms persist:

- PCI (stent)
- CABG

Key point

Stable angina = predictable exertional chest pain relieved by rest or GTN.

Unstable Angina

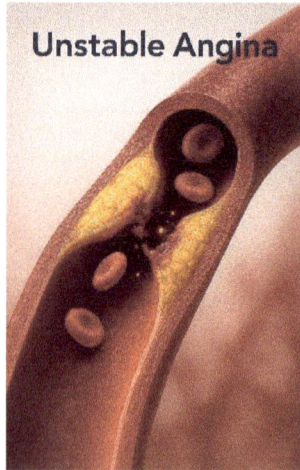

- Pain occurs at rest or worsening pattern
- Not reliably relieved by GTN
- Medical emergency

Common Symptoms

- Central chest pain radiating to arm, jaw, neck, or back
- Breathlessness
- Nausea, dizziness, anxiety

Stable angina is predictable and occurs with exertion, while unstable angina is unpredictable, occurs even at rest, lasts longer, and is a medical emergency.

Key Differences Between Stable and Unstable Angina

Feature	Stable Angina	Unstable Angina
Pattern	Predictable, follows a consistent pattern	Unpredictable, no clear pattern

Feature	Stable Angina	Unstable Angina
Triggers	Physical exertion, emotional stress, wintry weather, heavy meals	Can occur at rest, during sleep, or with minimal effort
Duration	Usually short (1–5 minutes, rarely >15 minutes)	Longer-lasting (>15–20 minutes, sometimes 30+ minutes)
Relief	Improves with rest or nitro-glycerine	May not improve with rest or medication
Severity	Less severe, manageable with lifestyle changes and medication	More severe, sudden worsening of symptoms
Urgency	Not usually an emergency, but requires medical follow-up	Always an emergency — immediate medical attention needed
Classification	Not part of acute coronary syndrome (ACS)	Classified as ACS (warning sign of a heart attack)
Cause	Narrowing of the coronary arteries due to plaque buildup	Plaque rupture and clot formation cause sudden reduced blood flow

Sources: Very well Health, Medicover Hospitals, Coppell ER

Why This Matters

- **Stable angina** is a chronic condition that can often be managed with medication, lifestyle changes, and monitoring.
- **Unstable angina** is a red flag for an impending heart attack. It reflects a sudden change in coronary artery disease and requires **emergency care**.

Quick Takeaway

If chest pain is **new, worsening, occurs at rest, lasts longer than usual, or does not improve with nitro-glycerine**, it should be treated as **unstable angina** and warrants **immediate emergency evaluation**.

12. Myocardial Infarction (Heart Attack)

A **heart attack**, medically called a **myocardial infarction (MI)**, happens when **blood flow to part of the heart muscle is suddenly blocked**, causing that portion of the heart muscle to be **damaged or die** due to lack of oxygen.

Main cause

The most common cause is **coronary artery disease**:

1. **Fatty plaques (atherosclerosis)** build up in the coronary arteries
2. A plaque **ruptures**
3. A **blood clot (thrombus)** forms on the rupture
4. The clot **blocks blood flow** to the heart muscle
5. The heart muscle downstream becomes **ischemic and necrotic**

What happens to the heart

- Oxygen deprivation begins within minutes
- Irreversible muscle damage can occur after **20–40 minutes**
- The affected heart muscle loses its ability to contract normally

Common symptoms

- Chest pain or pressure (often radiating to arm, jaw, or back)
- Shortness of breath
- Sweating, nausea, dizziness
- Fatigue (especially in women and older adults)

Illustration: cause of a heart attack

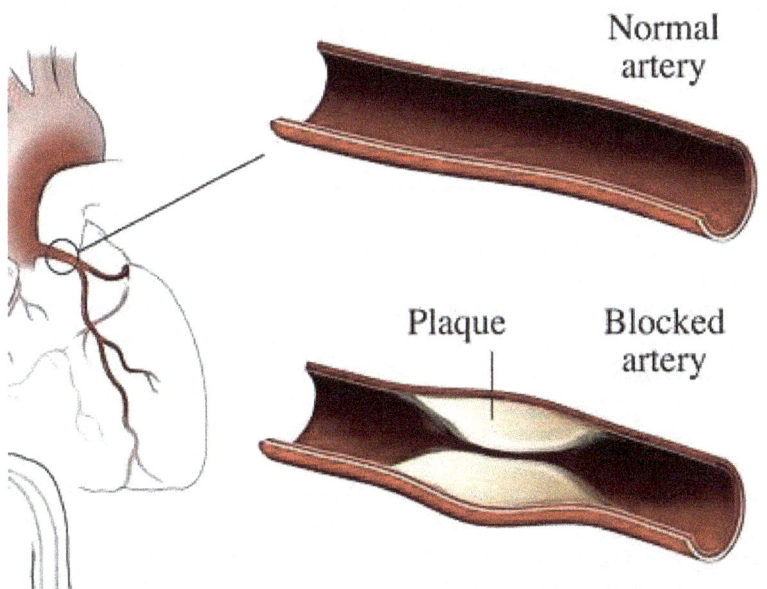

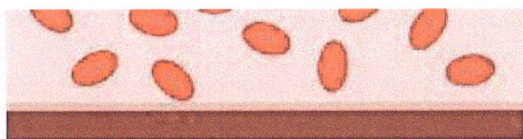

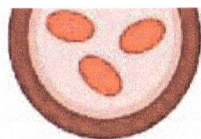

Normal artery

Plaque   Blocked artery

Plaque build-up

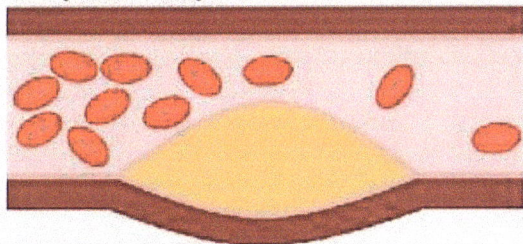

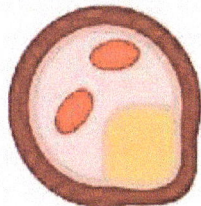

Plaque rupture

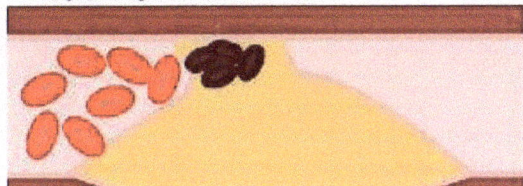

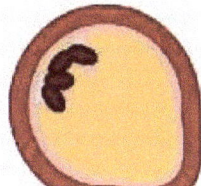

Key point to remember

A heart attack is **not** caused by the heart "stopping," but by **blocked blood supply** to the heart muscle.

STEMI vs NSTEMI (Types of Heart Attacks)

Both **STEMI** and **NSTEMI** are forms of **acute myocardial infarction (AMI)**, meaning heart muscle damage caused by reduced blood flow. The key difference lies in the **degree of coronary artery blockage and ECG findings**.

STEMI

ST-Elevation Myocardial Infarction

What happens

- **Complete (or near-complete) blockage** of a coronary artery
- Causes **full-thickness (transmural) myocardial infarction**

ECG findings

- **ST-segment elevation** in **≥2 contiguous leads**
- May later develop **pathologic Q waves**

Cardiac enzymes

- **Troponin: elevated**

Treatment urgency

Immediate reperfusion required

- Primary **PCI (angioplasty/stent)** preferred
- **Thrombolytics** if PCI unavailable
-

NSTEMI

Non-ST-Elevation Myocardial Infarction

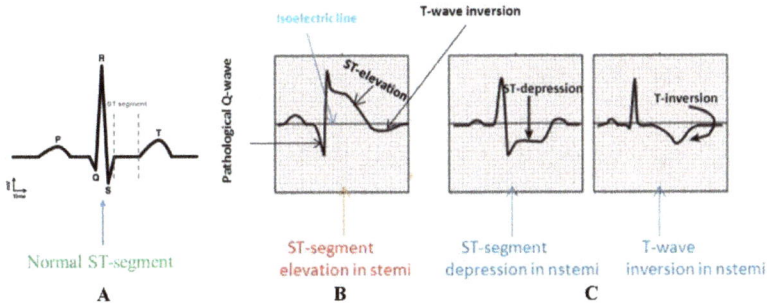

What happens

- **Partial or intermittent blockage** of a coronary artery
- Causes **partial-thickness (subendocardial) infarction**

ECG findings

- **No ST elevation**
- May show:
    - o **ST depression**
    - o **T-wave inversion**
    - o Or **normal ECG**

Cardiac enzymes

- **Troponin: elevated**

Treatment urgency

Urgent but not immediate reperfusion

- Antiplatelets, anticoagulants
- Early invasive strategy (angiography within 24–72 hrs)

STEMI-occurs when a coronary artery is completely blocked, leading to full-thickness heart muscle damage.
Myocardial Infarction Type 1

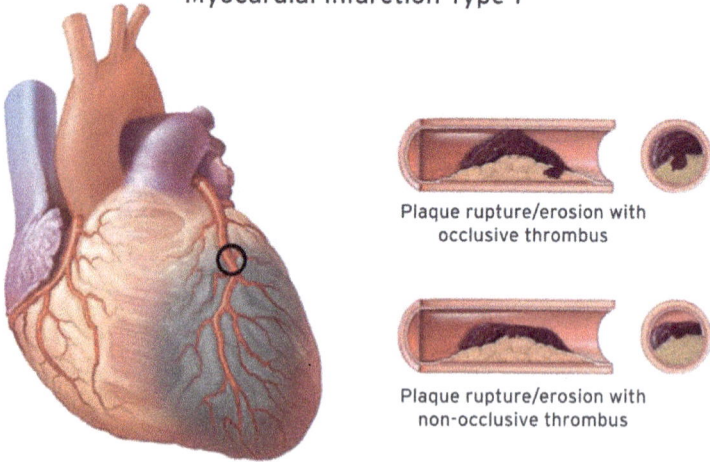

Plaque rupture/erosion with occlusive thrombus

Plaque rupture/erosion with non-occlusive thrombus

NSTEMI (Non–Non-ST-Elevation Myocardial Infarction)

NSTEMI is a type of **heart attack** in which there is **heart muscle damage due to reduced blood flow**, but **without ST-segment elevation on the ECG**.

What happens in NSTEMI

- A **coronary artery is partially or intermittently blocked**
- Blood flow is **reduced, not completely stopped**
- Causes **partial-thickness (subendocardial) damage** to the heart muscle

ECG findings

- **No ST elevation**
- May show:
    - **ST-segment depression**
    - **T-wave inversion**
    - Or even a **normal ECG**

Blood tests

- **Cardiac troponins: elevated** (confirms myocardial injury)

How NSTEMI differs from STEMI

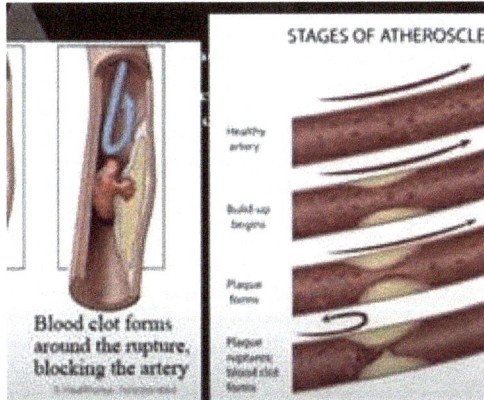

Feature	NSTEMI	STEMI
Artery blockage	Partial	Complete
ST elevation	✘ No	✓ Yes
Heart muscle damage	Partial thickness	Full thickness
Immediate PCI	Usually not immediate	Immediate

Key takeaway

NSTEMI = heart attack with elevated troponin but no ST elevation, usually due to partial coronary artery blockage.

Difference Between NSTEMI and Unstable Angina

Both **NSTEMI** and **unstable angina (UA)** are forms of **acute coronary syndrome (ACS)** and often look similar clinically. The **key difference** is **heart muscle damage**, which is identified by **cardiac troponin levels**.

NSTEMI (Non–ST-Elevation Myocardial Infarction)

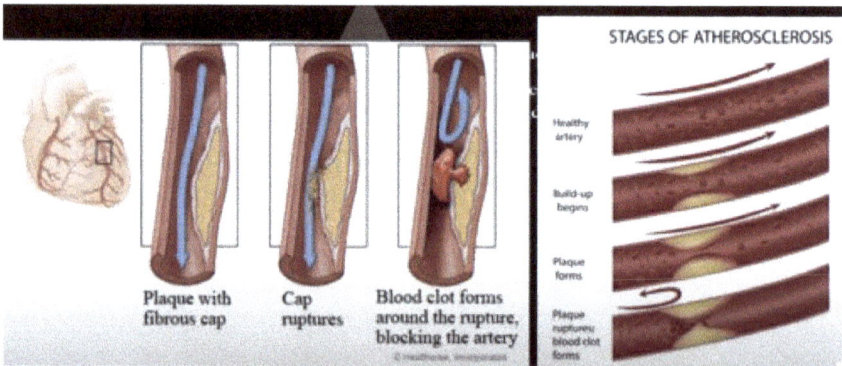

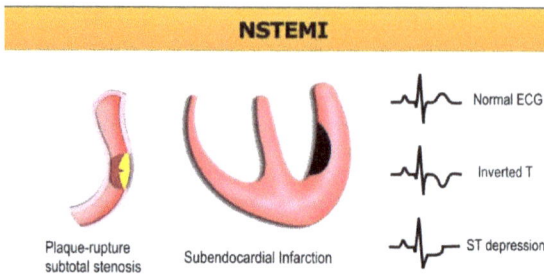

STAGES OF ATHEROSCLEROSIS

Healthy artery

Build-up begins

Plaque forms

Plaque ruptures, blood clot forms

Plaque with fibrous cap

Cap ruptures

Blood clot forms around the rupture, blocking the artery

NSTEMI

Plaque-rupture subtotal stenosis

Subendocardial Infarction

Normal ECG

Inverted T

ST depression

What happens

- **Partial or intermittent coronary artery blockage**
- Causes **irreversible myocardial cell death**

ECG

- No ST elevation
- May show **ST depression or T-wave inversion**

Troponin

- **Elevated** ✅

Unstable Angina and NSTEMI

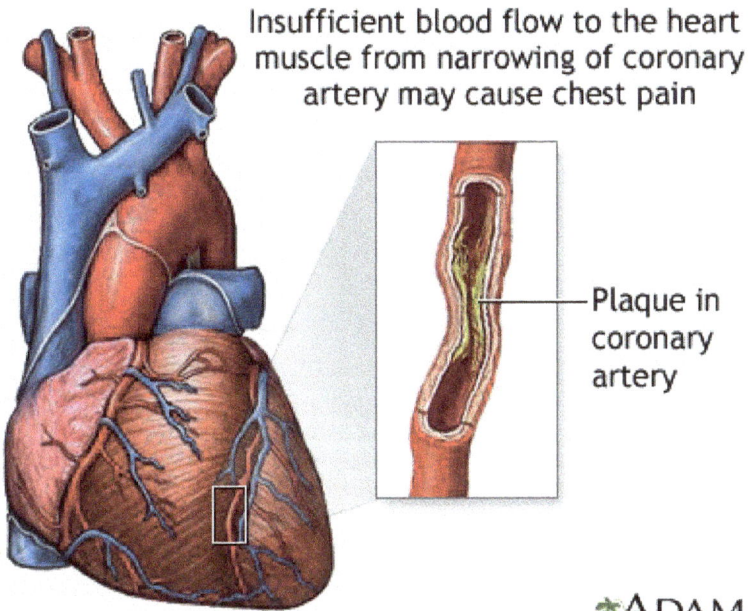

Insufficient blood flow to the heart muscle from narrowing of coronary artery may cause chest pain

Plaque in coronary artery

✻A.D.A.M.

What happens

- **Transient or incomplete ischemia**
- **No myocardial cell death**

ECG

- Normal or **transient ST depression/T-wave inversion**

Troponin

- **Normal**

Side-by-side comparison

Feature	NSTEMI	Unstable Angina
Coronary blockage	Partial	Partial/transient
Myocardial damage	✓ Yes (infarction)	✗ No

Feature	NSTEMI	Unstable Angina
Troponin	**Elevated**	**Normal**
ECG	ST ↓ / T inversion	Normal or transient changes
Prognosis	Worse than UA	Better than NSTEMI

High-yield clinical rule

Troponin elevated = NSTEMI

Troponin normal = Unstable angina

STEMI vs NSTEMI — Quick comparison

Feature	STEMI	NSTEMI
Coronary blockage	Complete	Partial
ST elevation on ECG	✓ Yes	✗ No
Troponin	Elevated	Elevated
Heart muscle damage	Full thickness	Partial thickness
Immediate PCI	✓ Required	✗ Not immediate

Clinical tip

ST elevation = total occlusion = immediate Cath lab

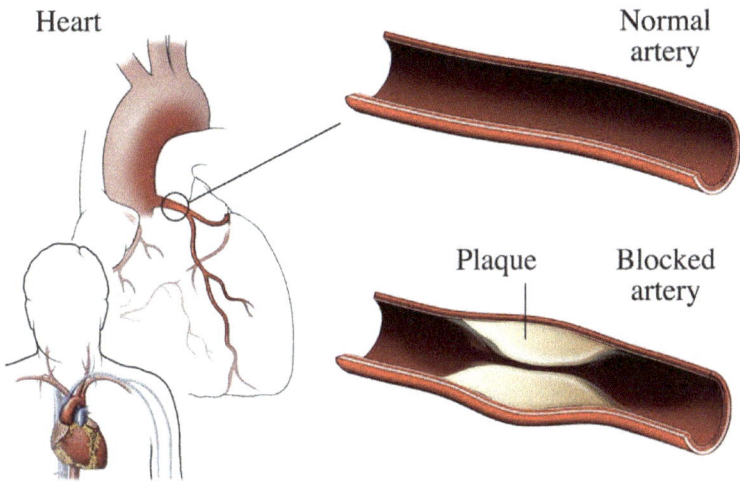

Heart

Normal artery

Plaque

Blocked artery

Occurs due to **coronary artery blockage**, leading to heart muscle death.

Symptoms

- Persistent crushing chest pain (>15 minutes)
- Breathlessness
- Nausea or vomiting
- Pale, clammy skin
- Sense of impending doom

13. Emergency Medications

Glyceryl Trinitrate (GTN)

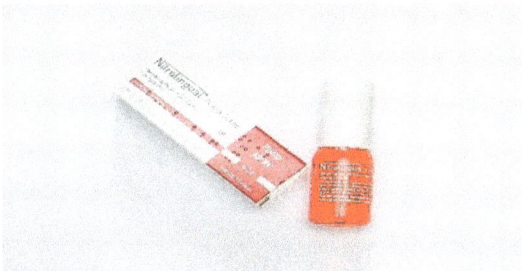

Indication: Suspected angina or MI if systolic BP ≥90 mmHg

- Spray: 400 micrograms sublingually
- Repeat every 5 minutes if required

Contraindications:

- Hypotension
- Recent PDE-5 inhibitors (e.g. sildenafil within 24–48h)
- Head injury or intracranial haemorrhage

Side effects: Headache, dizziness, hypotension

Aspirin

Indication: Suspected ACS

- Adult dose: **300 mg orally (chewed or dissolved)**

Do NOT give if:

- Known aspirin allergy
- Active GI bleeding

Caution (benefit usually outweighs risk):

- Asthma, pregnancy, renal disease

SUDDEN CARDIAC ARREST (SCA)

Sudden cardiac arrest occurs when the heart **abruptly stops pumping blood effectively**, leading to **loss of cardiac output, loss of consciousness, and absence of a pulse**. Without immediate treatment, it is **rapidly fatal**.

Survival

- Overall survival to hospital discharge in out-of-hospital cardiac arrest is **8–10%**
- Survival depends on:
    - **Early recognition**
    - **Immediate high-quality CPR**
    - **Early defibrillation (if shockable rhythm)**
    - **Rapid advanced life support and post-resuscitation care**

Chain of Prevention in a Dental Setting

1. Identify Risk Early

- Take a thorough medical history at every visit
- Identify high-risk patients (e.g. cardiac disease, diabetes, asthma, allergies)
- Reduce triggers: anxiety, pain, dehydration, prolonged supine positioning

2. Prepare the Team

- All staff trained in **BLS, AED use, and medical emergencies**
- Annual updates and regular practice drills
- Clear roles agreed in advance (who calls 999, who starts CPR, who gets the AED)

3. Prepare the Environment

- Emergency drugs and equipment immediately accessible

- AED available on site
- Oxygen, suction, airway equipment checked regularly and documented

4. Recognise Deterioration Early

- Use **ABCDE approach** for unwell patients
- Recognise red flags: collapse, unresponsiveness, abnormal breathing
- Act early — do not wait for cardiac arrest

5. Respond Immediately

- Call **999 or 112** early
- Start **high-quality CPR** if cardiac arrest is suspected
- Use the **AED as soon as it is available**
- Follow dispatcher instructions until help arrives

6. Review & Learn

- Handover clearly to ambulance crew
- Debrief the team after the event
- Update training, protocols, and equipment checks as needed

Good prevention = good preparation.

Early risk assessment, trained staff, ready equipment, and fast action save lives.

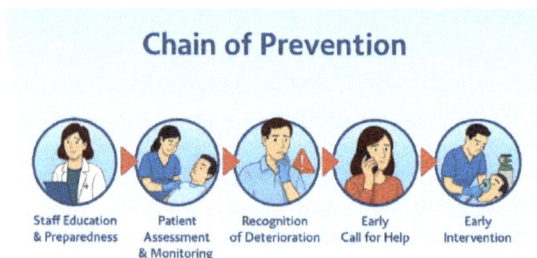

Chain of Prevention

Staff Education & Preparedness | Patient Assessment & Monitoring | Recognition of Deterioration | Early Call for Help | Early Intervention

CAUSES OF CARDIAC ARREST

According to the **Resuscitation Council UK (ALS)**, causes should be systematically considered using the **Reversible Causes: the 4 Hs and 4 Ts**.

The 4 Hs

Hypoxia

- Most common cause
- From airway obstruction, respiratory failure, asthma, pneumonia, opioid overdose

Hypovolaemia

- Severe blood or fluid loss
- Trauma, GI bleeding, dehydration, sepsis

Hypo-/Hyperkalaemia (and other metabolic disturbances)

- Electrolyte imbalance (especially potassium)
- Diabetic ketoacidosis (DKA)
- Renal failure

Hypothermia

- Core temperature <35°C
- Reduced cardiac excitability and contractility

The 4 Ts

Tension pneumothorax

- Air trapped under pressure in pleural space
- Compresses heart and lungs → obstructive shock

Cardiac tamponade

- Fluid/blood in pericardial sac
- Prevents ventricular filling

Toxins

- Drug overdose (opioids, TCAs, beta-blockers, calcium channel blockers)
- Poisoning

Thrombosis

- **Coronary thrombosis** → acute myocardial infarction
- **Pulmonary thrombosis** → massive pulmonary embolism

Common clinical conditions leading to cardiac arrest

(Integrated into Hs and Ts per guidelines)

- **Myocardial infarction** → Coronary thrombosis
- **Pulmonary embolism** → Pulmonary thrombosis
- **Diabetic ketoacidosis** → Metabolic disturbance (H)
- **Sepsis** → Hypovolaemia, hypoxia, metabolic acidosis
- **Severe asthma** → Hypoxia
- **Hypothermia** → Hypothermia (H)

Key NICE & RCUK principles

- Cardiac arrest management prioritises:
  - **Immediate CPR**
  - **Early defibrillation for shockable rhythms (VF/pVT)**
  - **Rapid identification and treatment of reversible causes**
- **Asystole and PEA are non-shockable rhythms**
- Treating the **underlying cause** is essential for survival

Summary

Sudden cardiac arrest = sudden loss of cardiac output

Think 4 Hs and 4 Ts

Early CPR and defibrillation save lives

Dental Resuscitation Equipment Requirements

Defibrillation Equipment

- **Automated External Defibrillator (AED)**
    - Must be **immediately accessible** in all clinical areas where patients are seen, including:
        - Dentists
        - Dental hygienists or therapists
        - Dental technicians (if treating patients)
        - Any combination of dental team members
- The AED must be:
    - Clearly visible
    - **Indicated with standard AED signage**
    - Checked regularly and maintained according to manufacturer instructions

Defibrillator Accessories

- **Adhesive defibrillator pads**
    - Adult pads (mandatory)
    - **Spare set of pads strongly recommended**
- **Scissors**
- **Razor** (for chest hair removal if required)

Emergency Drug Kit

- An **appropriate emergency drug kit** must be available **on-site** in dental practices where clinicians are permitted to administer medicines.

- Drugs should align with current **RCUK dental emergency recommendations** (e.g. for anaphylaxis, hypoglycaemia, asthma, cardiac arrest).
- Drugs must be:
  - In-date
  - Clearly labelled
  - Easily accessible
- Staff must be trained in:
  - Indications
  - Doses
  - Routes of administration

Oxygen and Airway Management Equipment

Oxygen Supply

- Each practice should have:
  - A **CD-size integral valve oxygen cylinder**
  - Capacity: **approximately 460 litres**
  - Capable of delivering:
    - **15 litres/minute**
    - For **approximately 30 minutes**
- Oxygen cylinders must be:
  - Securely stored
  - Regularly checked
  - Immediately available

Oxygen Delivery Equipment

- Oxygen tubing
- Oxygen masks with a reservoir
- Clear face masks compatible with self-inflating bags

Ventilation Equipment

- **Self-inflating bag with reservoir (adult)**
- **Self-inflating bag with reservoir (child)**
- **Clear face masks** for self-inflating bags:

- Sizes **0, 1, 2, 3, and 4**

Airway Adjuncts

Oropharyngeal airways

- A full set of **7 sizes**:
  - 000, 00, 0, 1, 2, 3, 4
- **Pocket face masks**
  - A set of **5 clear pocket masks**, sizes **1–5**
  - Must include an **oxygen port**
  - Available **immediately within the first minutes** of a cardiac arrest

Suction Equipment

- **Portable suction device**
  - Must be:
    - Immediately available
    - Functional
    - Suitable for clearing airway secretions during resuscitation

Personal Protective Equipment (PPE)

The following must be available **immediately** in the event of cardiac arrest:

- Gloves
- Aprons
- Eye protection

Dental Technicians (CDTs) – Regulatory Clarification

Under the **Human Medicines Regulations 2012**:

- **Clinical Dental Technicians (CDTs):**

- Are **not permitted** to purchase or hold **prescription-only medicines**
- Are **not required** to have an emergency drug kit
- Are **not expected** to be trained in the use of emergency drugs
- The **Care Quality Commission (CQC)** does **not expect**:
  - Independently working CDTs
  - Or CDT-only premises to hold emergency drugs on-site

Key Compliance Points (CQC & RCUK)

- Equipment must be:
  - Immediately accessible
  - Regularly checked and documented
- Staff must:
  - Receive **annual training** in basic life support
  - Be familiar with the location and use of all resuscitation equipment
- Practices should conduct:
  - Regular **emergency drills**
  - Routine audits of emergency equipment

CQC Inspection Checklist – Dental Resuscitation Equipment & Preparedness

Practice Name: _____

Practice Address: _____

Inspection / Audit Date: _____

Responsible Lead: _____

1. Defibrillation Equipment

☐ **AED available on-site**

☐ AED is **immediately accessible** in all clinical areas

☐ AED location is **clearly visible**

☐ **Standard AED signage** in place

AED Accessories

☐ Adult adhesive defibrillator pads present
☐ **Spare set of pads available**
☐ Pads **in date**
☐ Scissors available
☐ Razor available (for chest hair removal)

Maintenance

☐ AED checked regularly
☐ Battery status checked and functional
☐ Maintenance log completed and up to date

2. Emergency Drug Kit

(Not applicable to CDT-only practices)

☐ Emergency drug kit present on-site
☐ Drugs align with **RCUK dental emergency recommendations**
☐ Drugs clearly labelled
☐ All drugs **in date**
☐ Drugs stored securely and accessible
☐ Staff trained in indications and administration

3. Oxygen Supply

☐ CD-size integral valve oxygen cylinder available
☐ Cylinder capacity approx. **460 litres**
☐ Capable of delivering **15 L/min**
☐ Cylinder sufficiently full
☐ Oxygen cylinder securely stored
☐ Regular checks documented

4. Oxygen Delivery Equipment

☐ Oxygen tubing available
☐ Oxygen masks with reservoir available
☐ Equipment clean and functional

5. Ventilation Equipment

☐ Adult self-inflating bag with reservoir
☐ Child self-inflating bag with reservoir
☐ Bags and reservoirs intact and functional

Face Masks

☐ Clear face masks compatible with bag-valve device
☐ Sizes available: 0 ☐ 1 ☐ 2 ☐ 3 ☐ 4 ☐

6. Airway Adjuncts

☐ Oropharyngeal airway set available
☐ Full set of sizes present:

- ☐ 000
- ☐ 00
- ☐ 0
- ☐ 1
- ☐ 2
- ☐ 3
- ☐ 4

☐ Airway adjuncts clean and in good condition

7. Pocket Face Masks

☐ Pocket face masks immediately available
☐ Total of **5 masks** present

□ Sizes 1–5 available
□ Masks include **oxygen port**
□ Masks clean and functional

8. Suction Equipment

□ Portable suction device available
□ Suction immediately accessible
□ Device tested and functional
□ Suction catheters available
□ Maintenance checks documented

9. Personal Protective Equipment (PPE)

□ Gloves available
□ Aprons available
□ Eye protection available
□ PPE immediately accessible during emergencies

10. Staff Training & Awareness

□ All clinical staff trained in **Basic Life Support (BLS)**
□ Training updated **annually**
□ Staff trained in use of AED
□ Staff aware of location of resuscitation equipment
□ Emergency drills conducted
□ Training records available

11. Dental Technicians (CDTs) – Regulatory Compliance

□ CDT-only practice identified (if applicable)
□ No prescription-only medicines held by CDTs
□ Emergency drug kit **not required** for CDT-only practices
□ Staff aware of scope of practice limitations

12. Documentation & Governance

☐ Emergency equipment checklist completed regularly
☐ Equipment checks documented
☐ Expiry dates monitored
☐ Policies align with **RCUK & NICE guidance**
☐ Evidence available for CQC inspection

Inspector / Auditor Comments

_____
_____
_____
_____

Action Plan (if required)

Issue Identified Action Required Responsible Person Target Date

Audit Outcome

☐ Fully compliant
☐ Partially compliant (action required)
☐ Non-compliant (urgent action required)

Auditor Name & Signature: _____
Date: _____

AIRWAY MANAGEMENT

OROPHARYNGEAL AIRWAY

Why OPA sizing matters

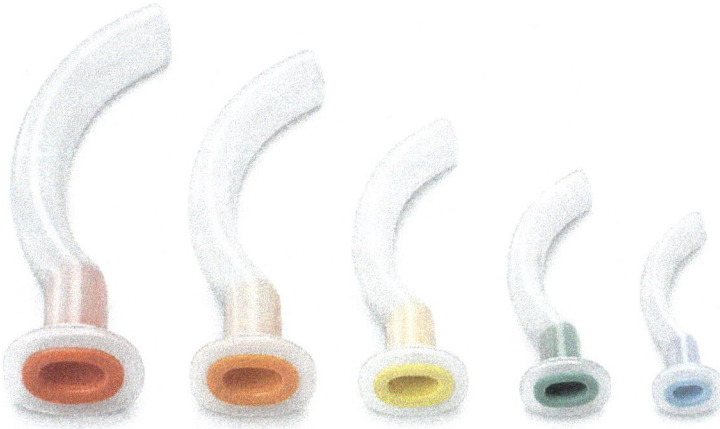

Choosing the right size of the OPA matters because the wrong size can obstruct the airway or cause injury:

Too small: Pushes the tongue backwards, worsening obstruction

Too large: presses on the epiglottis, gagging, trauma, vomiting

Correct size: keeps the airway open, allows ventilation, and allows effective airway management

THE SIZING METHODS

Corner of the mouth to angle of the Jaw

Or from incisors to the earlobe

INSERTING THE OPA

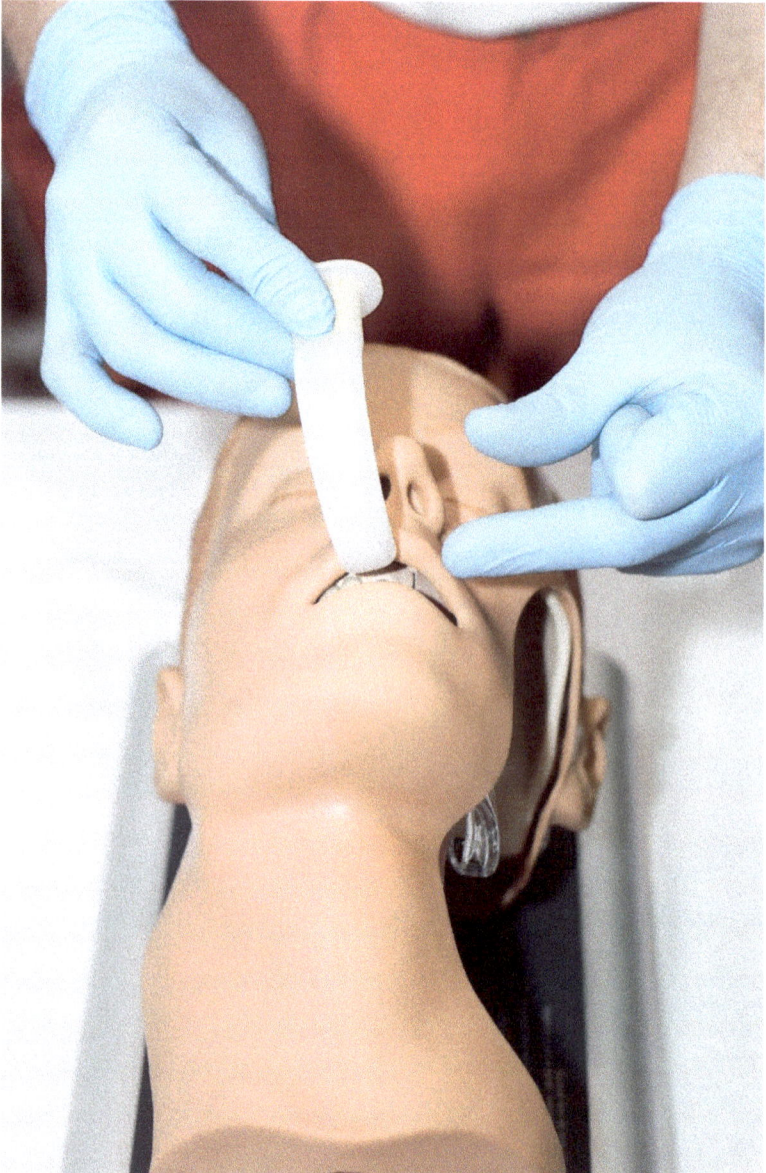

CARDIOPULMONARY RESUSCITATION (CPR)

Core Principles of CPR (All Ages)

- Ensure **safety** of rescuer and casualty
- **Early recognition** of cardiac arrest
- **Early CPR**
- **Early defibrillation**
- **Early advanced care**

If unresponsive and not breathing normally → start CPR immediately and send for a defibrillator.

ADULT CPR

Ensure the scene is safe for you and the casualty.

CHECK IF THE PATIENT IS RESPONSIVE

Kneel beside him.

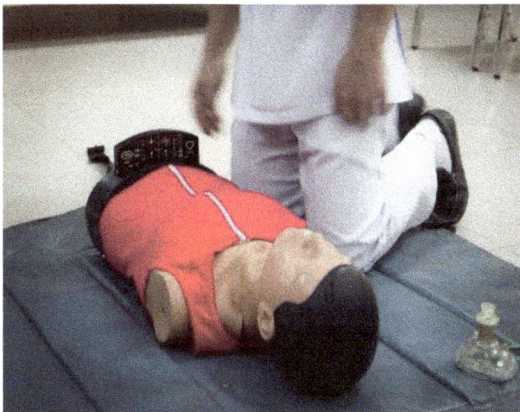

SHAKE THE PATIENT'S SHOULDER OR SQUEEZE THE EARLOBES OR THE TRAPEZIUS MUSCLES

Check whether the casualty is responsive by shaking the casualty's shoulder, speaking to the casualty, and saying, "Wake up!" "Squeeze my hand, squeeze the ear lobes, or press the supraorbital notch or the trapezius muscle.

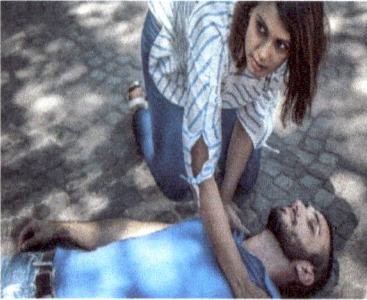

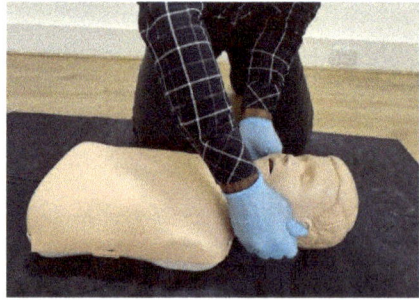

CALL 999/112 OR ASK A BYSTANDER TO CALL IF THE PATIENT IS UNRESPONSIVE. CALL 2222 IF IN THE HOSPITAL.

If unresponsive, proceed immediately to emergency call. Call first before checking breathing; call handlers will assist with breathing assessment.

⬚ Ask for an **ambulance and AED**.

⬚ If alone, use hands-free speaker or phone headset.

⬚ Dispatchers will help assess and guide CPR.

Give your location, your name, the names of the casualty, and the patient's condition. Ask for oxygen, a defibrillator, and any other resources you require to assist you in conducting adequate resuscitation.

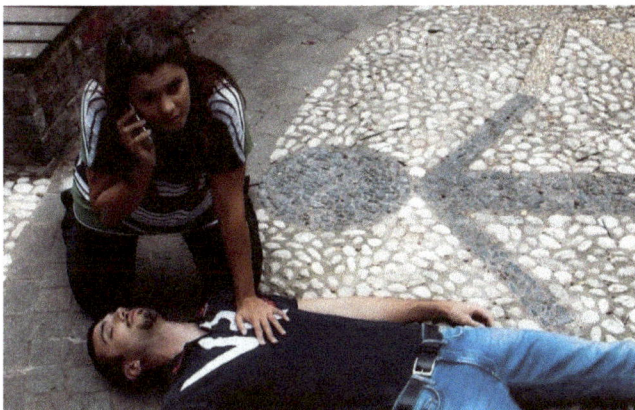

.Place one hand on the forehead.

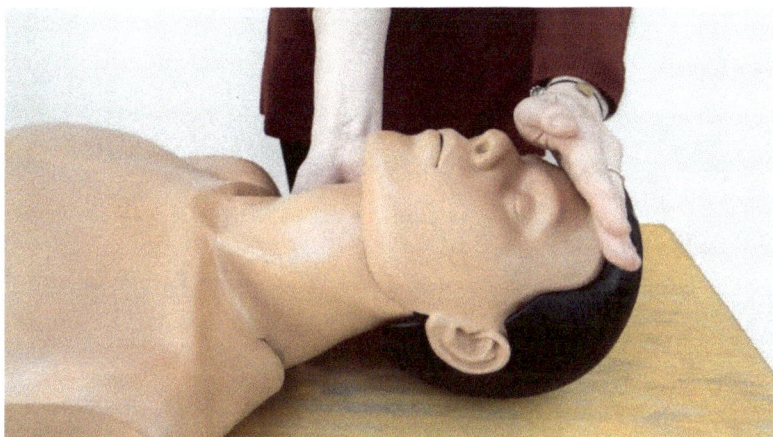

DO A HEAD TILT, CHIN LIFT

To maintain a clear airway, do a head tilt and chin lift. This will elevate the patient's relaxed tongue from the back of the airway to the front of the mouth. To achieve this, place your hand on your forehead, then lift your chin with the other hand.

ASSESS BREATHING

- Lower your head close to the casualty's face with your cheek close to the nose so that you can listen for any breath from the casualty's nose, feel the air from the casualty's nose on your cheek, and see the casualty's chest rise and fall. Do this for no more than 10 seconds. If the Casualty is **not breathing normally**, or breathing is **abnormal (agonal gasps)** assume cardiac arrest.

- **Do NOT delay CPR by over-analysing breathing patterns**.

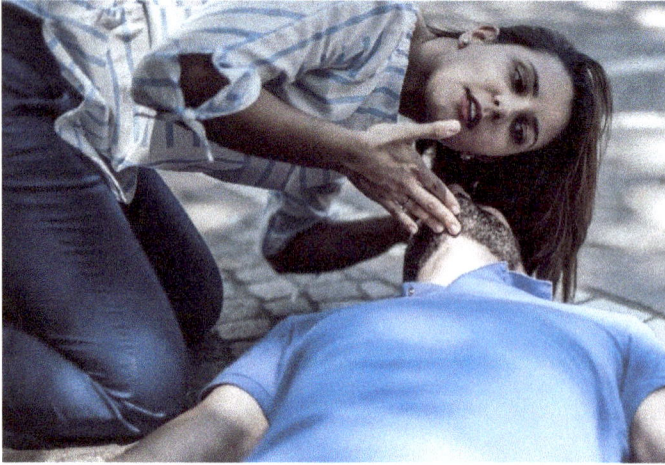

Start CPR Immediately

Chest Compressions

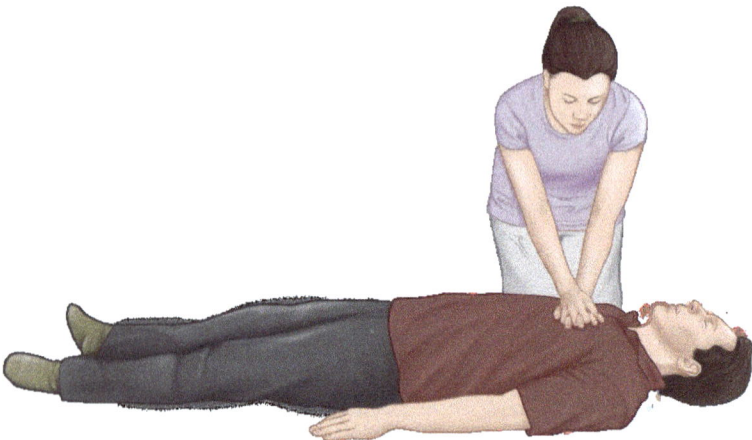

- Hand position: **centre of chest**
- Interlock fingers
- Arms straight, shoulders over hands

- Depth: **5–6 cm**
- Rate: **100–120 per minute**
- Allow **full chest recoil**

Compression–Ventilation Ratio

Conduct chest compressions immediately. For an adult, the ratio of compressions to breath should be thirty to two rescue breaths at 100-120 compressions per minute. On average, you are giving two compressions per second.

30 compressions : 2 breaths

Minimise interruptions

Continue until professional help arrives or AED prompts otherwise.

- Place the heel of your hand in the centre of the patient's Chest slightly above the tip of the breastbone. The position of your hand on the chest is vital to effective CPR.
- Place the second hand on top of the first hand, which is already positioned on the chest. Interlock your fingers and give thirty compressions at a rate of two compressions per second.
- 100-120 compressions per minute. Make sure your arms are straight and leaning slightly over the patient.
- Press down on the casualty's chest to a depth of 5-6cm.
- Release your pressure on the chest and watch it recoil before pressing down on the chest again.

Rescue breaths

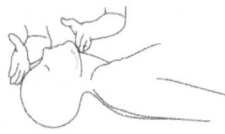

Open airways by
lifting the chin
slightly

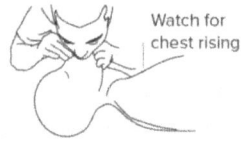

Watch for
chest rising

Pinch nose and give
two rescue breaths

Rescue Breaths

- **If trained and willing**:
  30 compressions : 2 breaths.
- **If untrained or unwilling to give breaths**:
  Continue **chest-compression-only CPR** guided by dispatcher.

Rescue Breath-Mouth-to-Mouth.

Seal your mouth over the patient's mouth while pinching their nose with your fingers. Keep the head tilted back to maintain an open airway. Only give mouth-to-mouth if you are confident there is no infection risk to you or the patient; if unsure, perform compression-only **CPR**.

Give **two rescue breaths**, each lasting about **one second**.

If you are unwilling or unable to give breaths, continue with **compression-only CPR**.

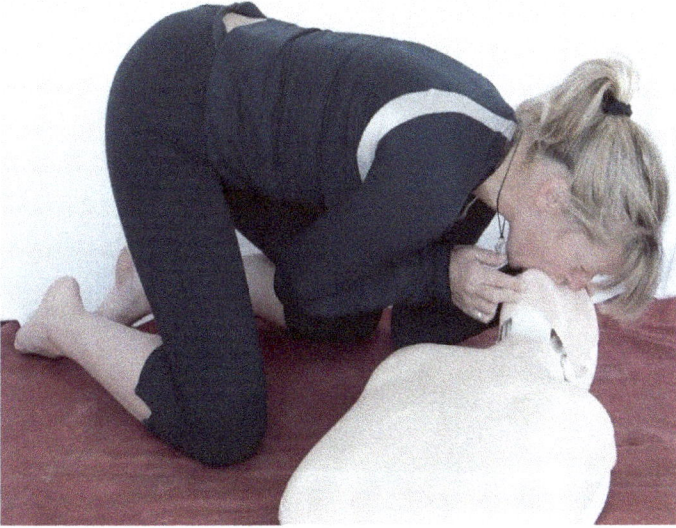

Rescue Breath-Mouth to face shield.

If you have a face shield, use it to minimise the risk of infection for you or the patient.

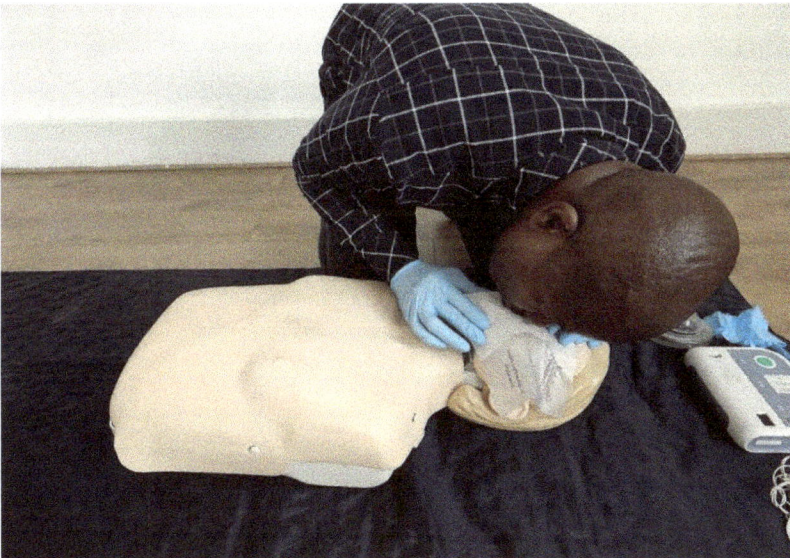

Rescue Breath- Mouth-to-Pocket Mask

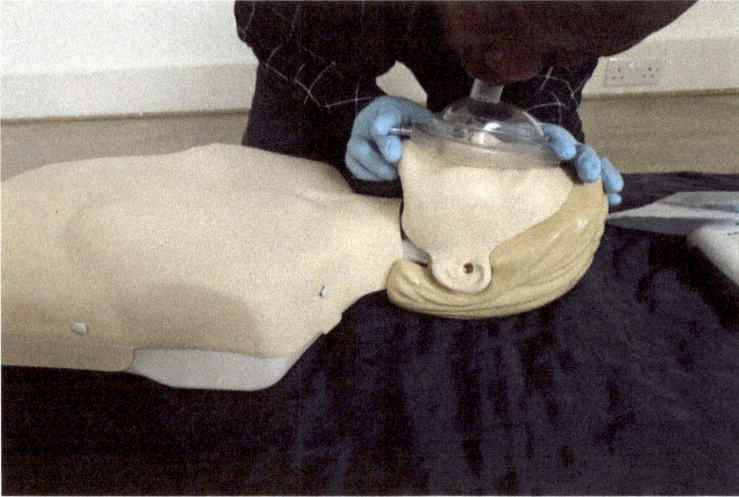

Rescue breathing can also be administered through a pocket Mask. This is another way of minimising the risk of infection.

Rescue Breath

Mouth-to-Bag Valve Mask (One-Person Technique)

One or two helpers can use a bag-valve mask (BVM). For a single-helpers technique, place one hand in a C-shape to seal the mask and

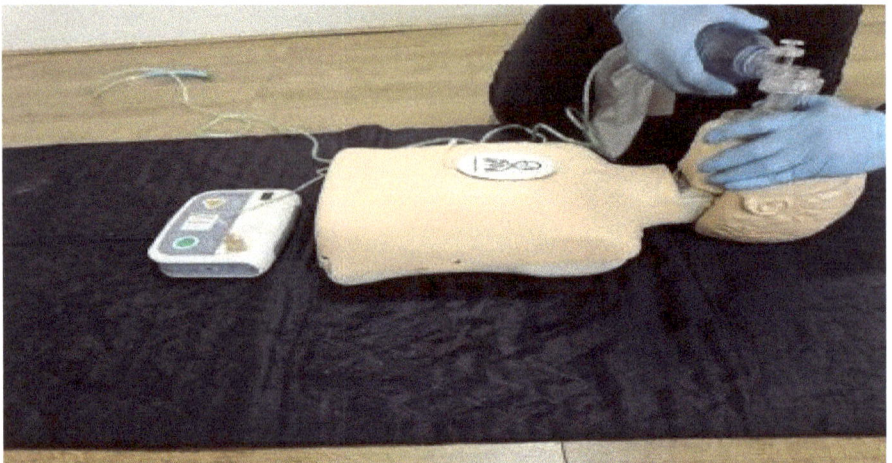

use the other hand in an E-shape to maintain head tilt. Squeeze the bag to deliver breaths.

Mouth-to-Bag Valve Mask—Two Persons Technique.

With both hands, one helper seals the BVM mask over the patient's nose and mouth while the other helper presses the oxygen bag to release the oxygen.

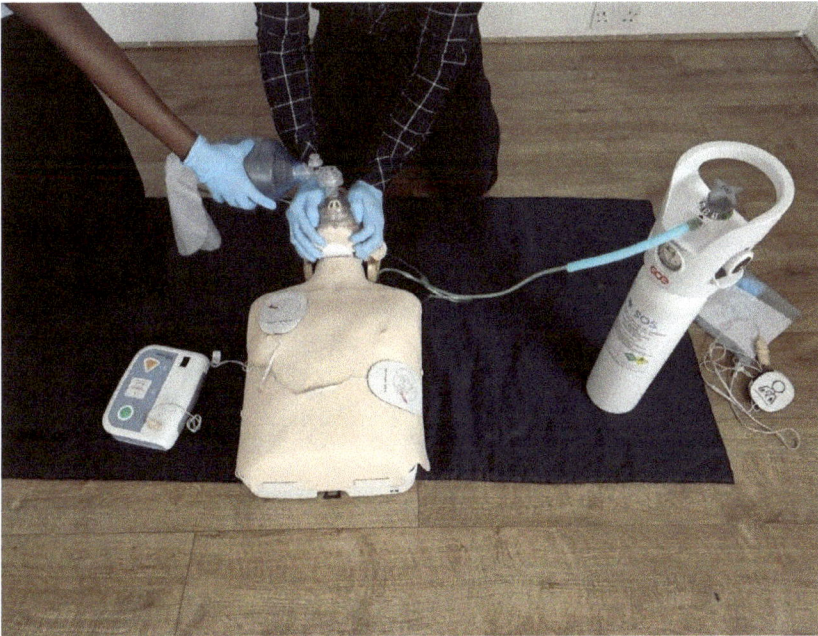

5) Use an AED (Automated External Defibrillator)

1. **Turn on AED as soon as available**
2. **Attach pads** to bare chest as shown on the pads
   - One pad on the **upper right chest**
   - One pad on the **left side below the armpit** (mid-axillary line)
3. Follow **voice prompts**.
4. **Deliver shock if advised**, then **resume CPR immediately**.

5. If three shocks fail, consider **changing pad position** (e.g., move the right-shoulder pad toward the centre of the chest to improve current flow) if trained.

6) Continue High-Quality CPR

- Continue CPR and AED cycles until:
  - **Signs of life return** (movement, normal breathing),
  - **Advanced responders take over**,
  - Or **you are unable to continue** due to exhaustion.

Special Considerations

If the arrest is due to drowning

→ Give **5 initial rescue breaths** before starting compressions, as hypoxia is the primary cause of arrest in these cases.

Vomiting or airway obstruction

✓ Ensure airway is clear
✓ Continue CPR with breaths if trained

SPECIAL SITUATION: CPR IN LATE PREGNANCY

When performing CPR on a heavily pregnant woman, raise the right hip slightly so that the pregnant woman is leaning slightly to the left side. This has the effect of moving the uterus away from the blood vessel and creating an uninterrupted blood supply to the heart.

PREGNANT WOMEN & CPR

Unconscious and Breathing place her on her left side
(Labour Left)

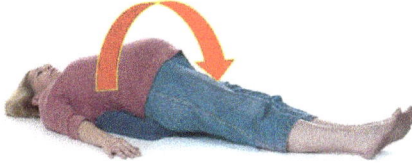

CPR in a **pregnant woman** should be done in cycles of 30 compressions **and** two breaths. It is also safe to use an automated external defibrillator, or AED, if one is available.

CHILD CPR (1 year to puberty)

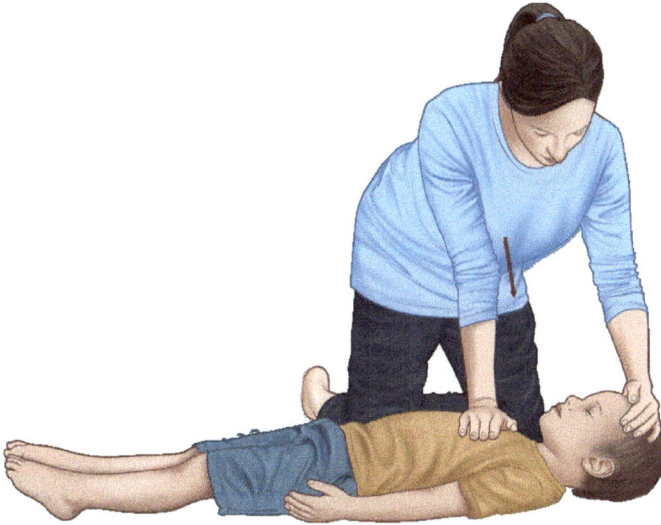

Key Differences

- Cardiac arrest is often **hypoxic**
- Rescue breaths are critical

Sequence

1. Danger
2. Response
3. Airway

4. Breathing
5. **5 initial rescue breaths**

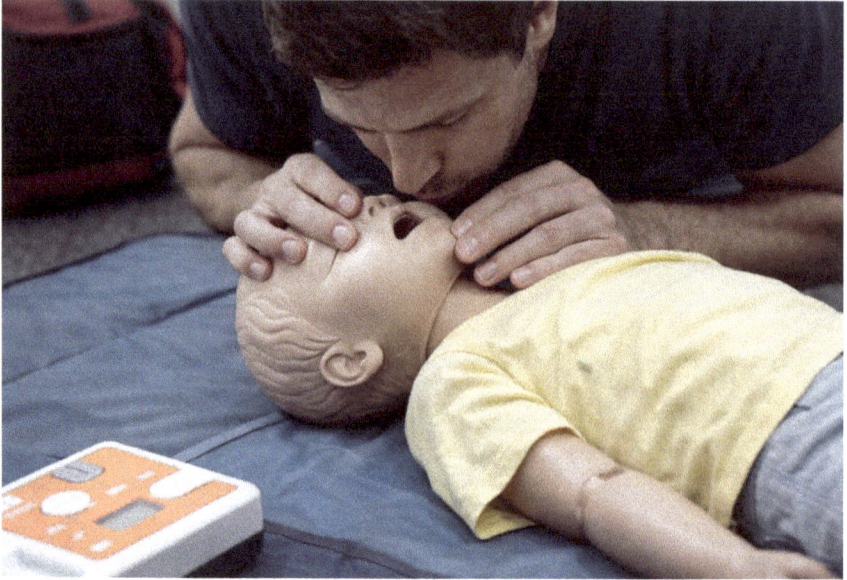

Chest Compressions

- One hand (or two for a larger child)
- Centre of chest
- Depth: **⅓ of chest**
- Rate: **100–120 per minute**

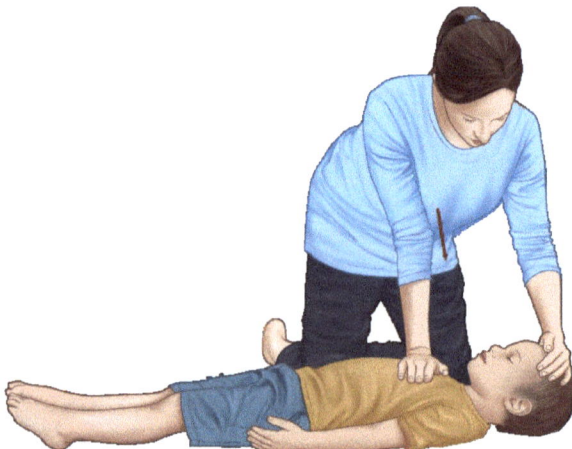

Compression–Ventilation Ratios

- **Healthcare professionals with paediatric duty:
  15 compressions: 2 breaths**
- **Bystanders & most clinicians:
  30 compressions: 2 breaths**

Defibrillation

- Use AED immediately
- Use **paediatric pads** if available
- If pads touch → **front-and-back placement**

INFANT CPR (<1 year)

Response

- Tickle feet
- Observe for movement or sound

Call 999 or 112

Airway

- Neutral head position
- **One finger** chin lift only

Breathing

Give **five rescue breaths**

- Mouth-to-mouth

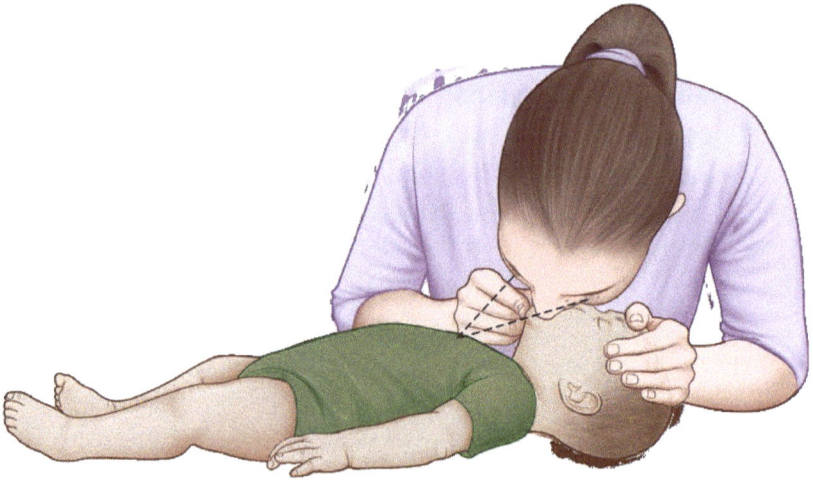

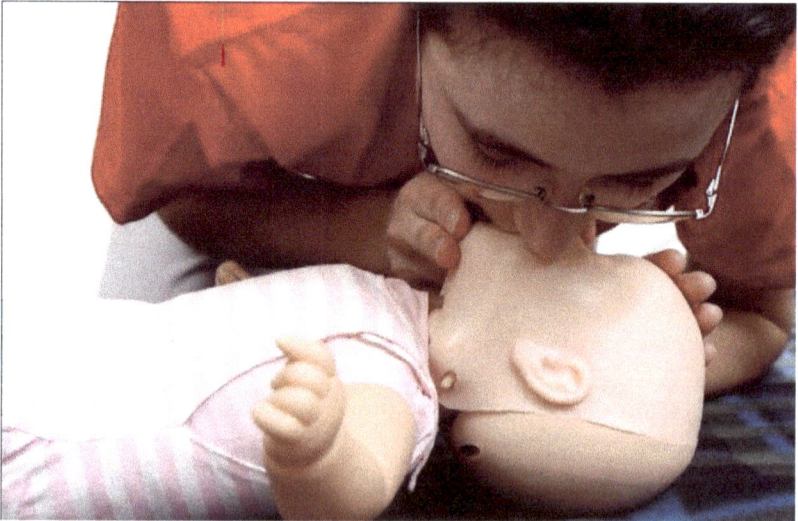

- Or mouth-to-nose if mouth injured
- Mouth to bag valve mask

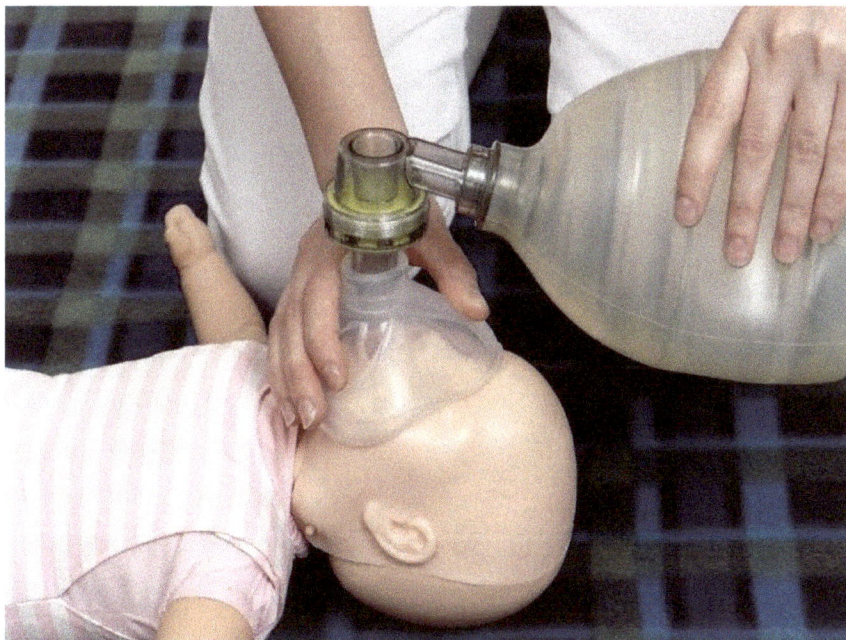

Chest Compressions

- Depth: ⅓ **of chest**

Ratios

- **Healthcare professionals with paediatric duty:
  15:2**
- **Bystanders:
  30:2**

Defibrillation

- Use AED as soon as available
- Use paediatric pads if possible
- Pad placement: **front and back**

- Infant compressions with two thumbs

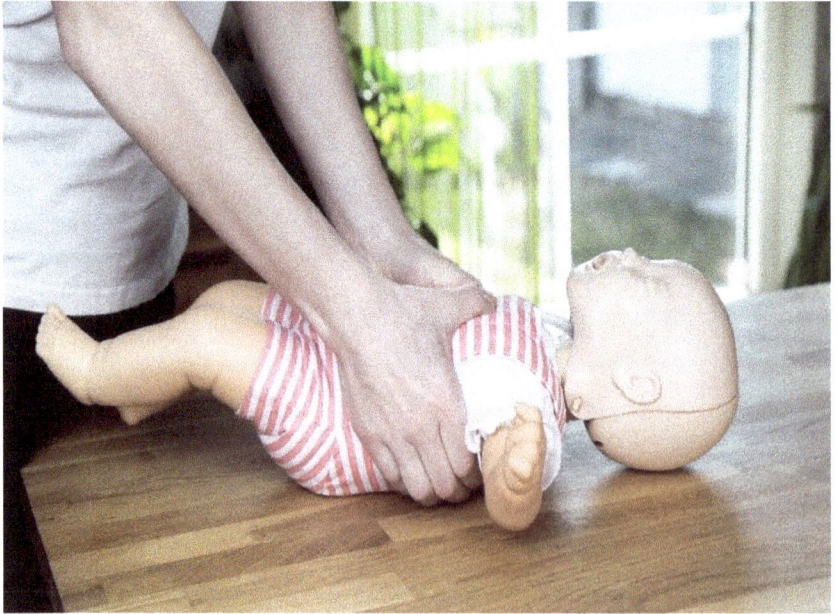

Fig 3. **Chest compression in infants: two-thumb encircling technique**

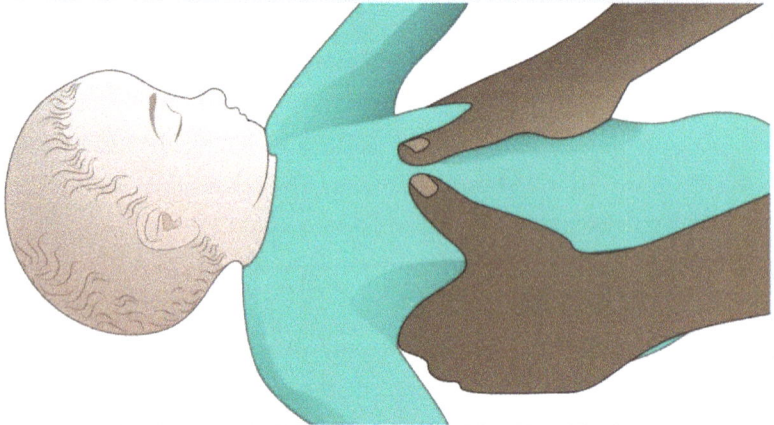

The two-thumb circling technique should be done with the thumbs side by side, and the hands encircling the infant's rib cage

DEFIBRILLATION

Key determinants of successful defibrillation:

- **Time to shock** – earlier defibrillation increases success

- **High-quality CPR** – before and between shocks maintains myocardial perfusion
- **Shockable rhythm** – VF and pulseless VT only
- **Myocardial condition** – oxygenation, perfusion, pH, and electrolytes
- **Correct energy & biphasic waveform**
- **Good pad position & contact** – low transthoracic impedance
- **Underlying cause** – primary cardiac causes respond best

DEFIBRILLATOR SIGNAGE

Every dental practice must have a defibrillator, and staff must know where it is located. The defibrillator signage must be properly displayed and visible to all members of staff and visitors to the practice.

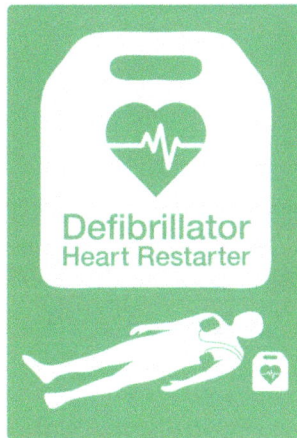

WHAT TO DO WHEN THE AED ARRIVES

Turn the machine on by pushing the on button. For most AEDs, the button will be green.

Making sure the casualty is bare-chested must be the case for all casualties, whether male or female, adult, or child. For female casualties, remove any bra and, if necessary, use scissors to cut through it.

Remove the electrodes or PADS from their seal and remove the backing paper to reveal the sticky part of the pads.

A defibrillator is a device that sends an electric shock to the heart to restore a normal heartbeat.

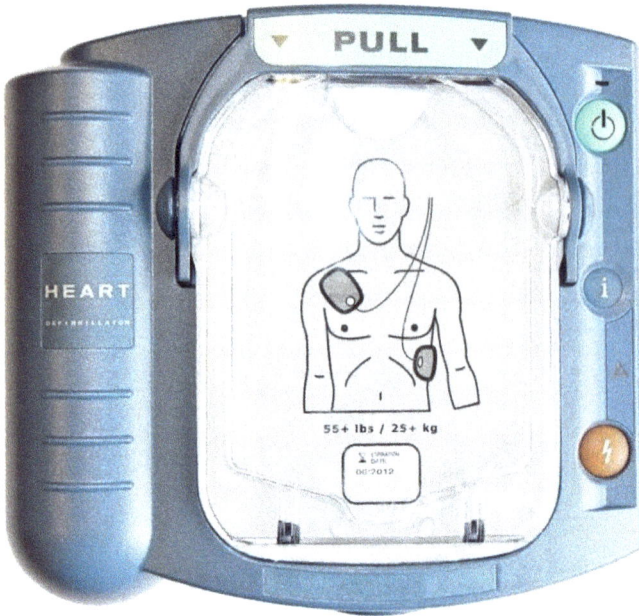

Steps for Using the AED

• When the AED arrives, turn the start button on, and it will automatically begin to issue instructions.

• Attach the electrode pads to the patient's bare chest.

• The AED will begin analysing the patient's heart rhythm. Do not touch the patient while the heart rhythm is being explored.

• If you have a semi-automatic defibrillator, it will ask you to press the shock button to deliver a shock if it detects a shockable rhythm.

Aftershock is delivered, and the AED will instruct you to continue CPR.

Common types of automated external defibrillators.

DEFIBRILLATOR SIGNAGE

Every dental practice must have a defibrillator, and staff must know where it is located. The defibrillator signage must be displayed appropriately and be visible to all staff and visitors to the practice.

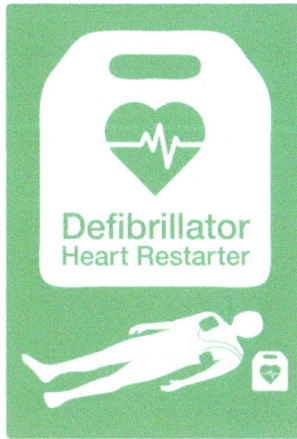

ATTACHING THE PADS

ANTERO-LATERAL PAD PLACEMENT

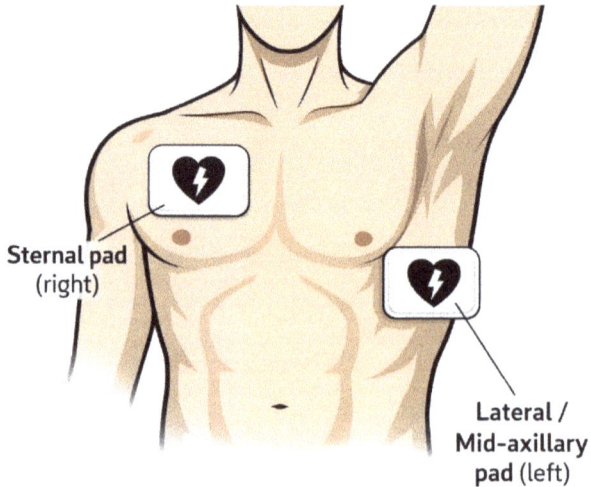

Sternal pad
(right)

Lateral /
Mid-axillary
pad (left)

Adult AED Pad Placement (Anterior–Lateral)

Correct pad placement is essential to ensure effective defibrillation by allowing electrical current to pass through the myocardium.

Anterior (Sternal) Pad – Adult

- Place one pad on the **right upper chest**
- Position it **just below the right clavicle**
- Ensure it is **to the right of the sternum**

Lateral (Apical) Pad – Adult

- Place the second pad on the **left side of the chest**
- Position it **below the left armpit (axilla)**
- Align it with the **mid-axillary line**, level with the lower edge of the pectoral muscle (approximately over the cardiac apex)

Rationale for Anterior–Lateral Pad Placement

This pad configuration:

- Allows the defibrillation current to pass **diagonally through the heart**
- Maximises the likelihood of successful defibrillation
- Prevents pad overlap
- Keeps pads clear of excessive breast tissue, muscle mass, and implanted devices (where possible)

Pads should always be applied **exactly as shown on the AED diagrams** when available.[29]

Key Clinical Points for Practice

- Remove excessive chest hair if pads will not adhere
- Ensure the chest is dry before pad application
- Do not delay defibrillation for pad repositioning unless placement is clearly incorrect
- Continue CPR immediately after shock delivery or if no shock is advised

References

29. Resuscitation Council UK. *Defibrillation and Automated External Defibrillators (AEDs) – Adult Basic Life Support*
30. European Resuscitation Council. *Guidelines for Resuscitation: Defibrillation*

Anteroposterior (AP) AED Pad Placement – Anterior Pad (Adult)

Anterior (Front) Pad

- Place the pad on the **left side of the chest**, over the **precordial area**
- Position it **to the left of the sternum**, overlying the heart
- **Do not place directly over the centre of the chest (sternum)**

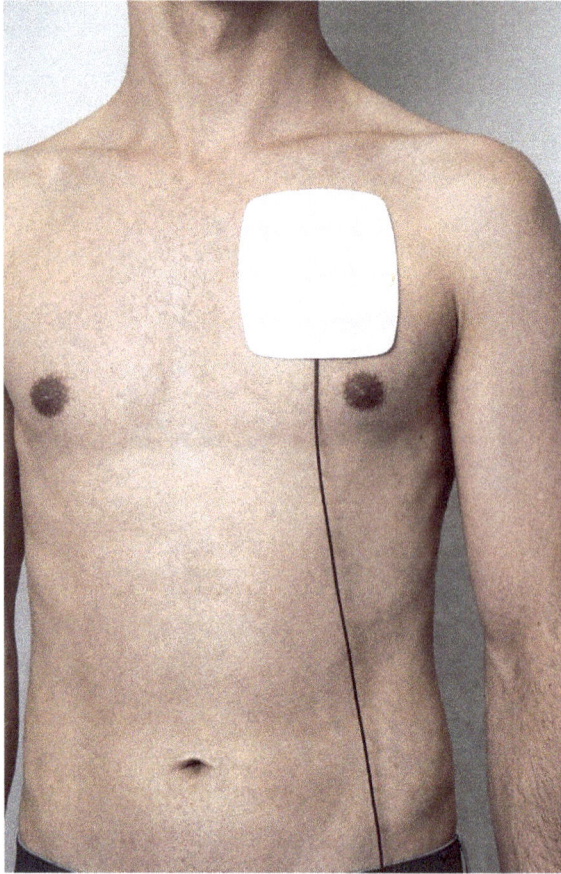

BACK(POSTERIOR) PAD

- Place the pad on the left side of the back
- Put it just below the left shoulder blade
- This pad is behind the heart

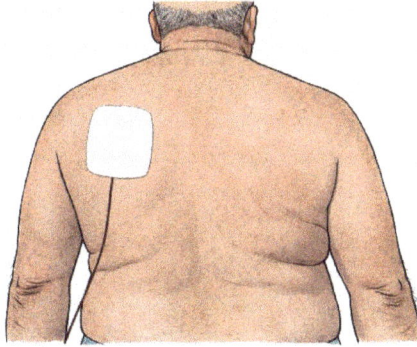

CHILD CPR- DEFIBRILLATING A CHILD- FRONT AND BACK PAD PLACEMENT.

1-12 years Front-Back

- Place the pads in the centre of the chest
- Position it between the nipples
- Back (posterior) pad
- Place on the centre of the back
- Position it between the shoulder blades

The goal is to have one pad on the chest and one on the back, with the heart between them.

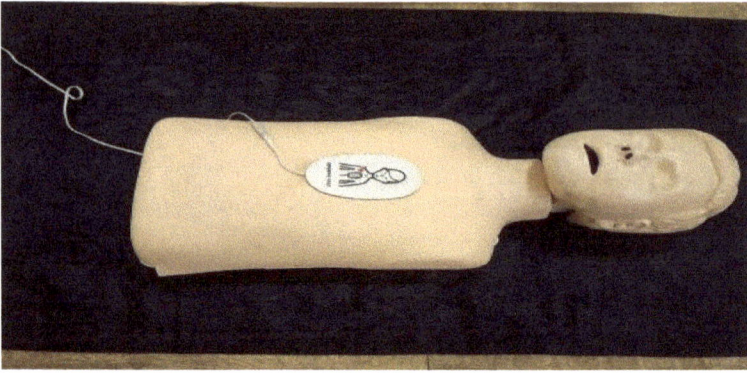

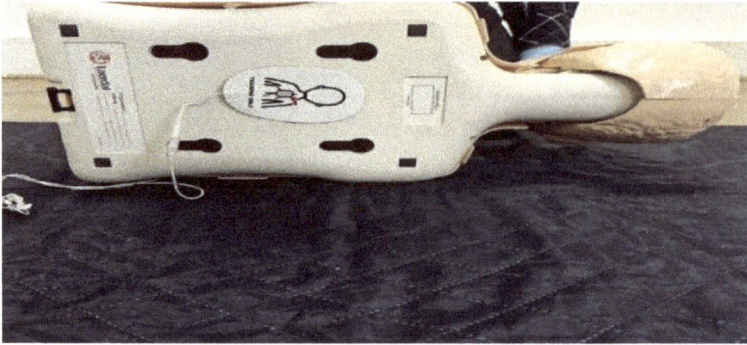

CHILD 13-18 YEARS – (ADOLESCENT) SAME AS ADULT

One pad on the upper right chest, and the other on the left side of the chest under the armpit.

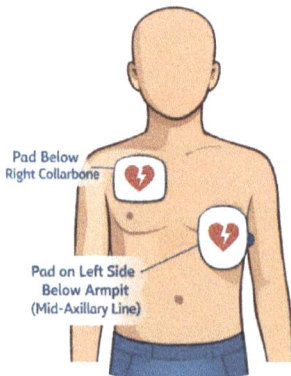

AED Pad Placement for Teen

Pad Below Right Collarbone

Pad on Left Side Below Armpit (Mid-Axillary Line)

HOW THE AED WORKS

- The pads have sensors called electrodes. When attached to the patient's chest, it sends information about the patient's heart rhythm to the AED's computer. The computer analyses the heart's rhythm to confirm whether a shock is necessary and, if required, will send a shock to correct the abnormal heart rhythm

TYPES OF DEFIBRILLATORS

- Automated External Defibrillators (AEDs)
- Implantable Cardioverter Defibrillators (ICDs)- surgically placed inside the body.

- Wearable Cardioverter Defibrillators (WCDs)-this rests on the body

SAFETY CONSIDERATIONS

JEWELLERY- remove pieces of jewellery and avoid placing the pads on them

MEDICATIONS- Do not place the pads on the pacemaker.

//**CLOTHING**- The patient must be bare-chested.

WATER/SWEAT-wipe any water

MEDICATIONS do not place pads on the GTN patch.

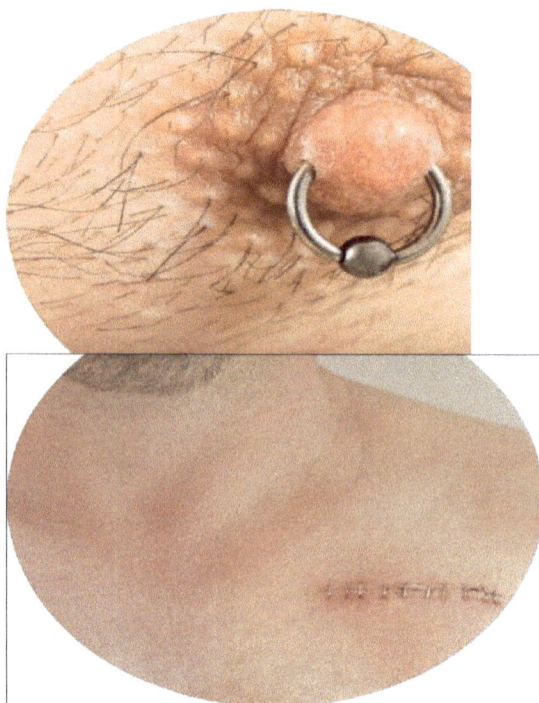

RESCUE BREATH METHODS (All Ages)

- Mouth-to-mouth
- Mouth-to-mask (preferred)
- Bag-Valve-Mask (BVM)
  - One-person: **C-E grip**
  - Two-person: One seals mask, one squeezes bag
- Mouth-to-nose (facial trauma)
- Mouth-to-stoma or tracheostomy (ventilate directly via stoma)

WHEN TO USE 15:2 IN CHILDREN

15:2

- Paediatric doctors & nurses
- Paramedics
- Emergency department staff

30:2

- Members of the public
- Dentists, GPs, school nurses
- Lone responders

Rationale: Simplicity and likelihood of adult CPR scenarios

RECOVERY POSITION (Breathing but Unresponsive adult)

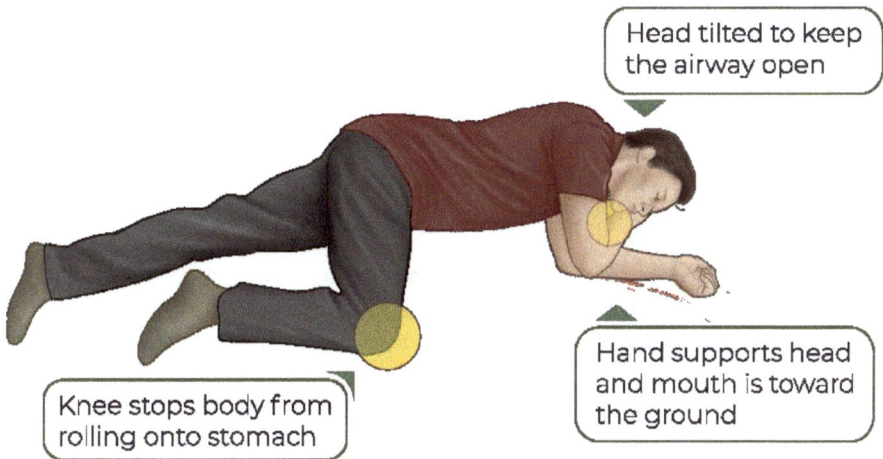

Head tilted to keep the airway open

Hand supports head and mouth is toward the ground

Knee stops body from rolling onto stomach

- Place in **lateral position**
- Head tilted, airway open
- Monitor breathing continuously

CHILD RECOVERY POSITION

CHECK FOR DANGER

Make sure you and the patient are safe.

CHECK FOR RESPONSIVENESS

Check whether the patient responds to a painful stimulus by squeezing the earlobes.

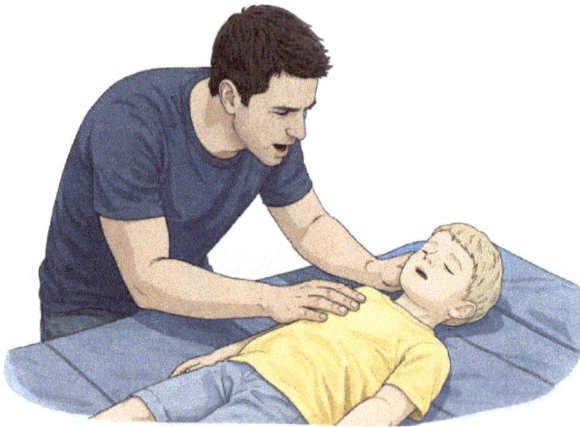

CHILD HEAD TILT, CHIN LIFT

Place one hand on the forehead and two fingers on the chin, tilt your head, and lift your chin.

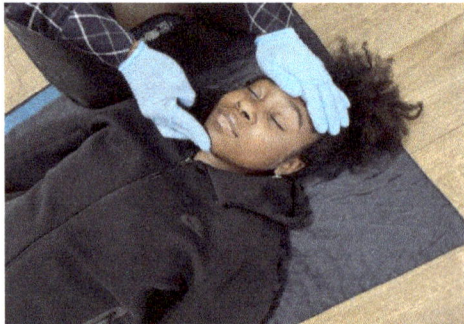

CHECK IF THE CHILD IS BREATHING

Lean towards the head with your cheek facing the casualty's nose to feel for the child's breath.

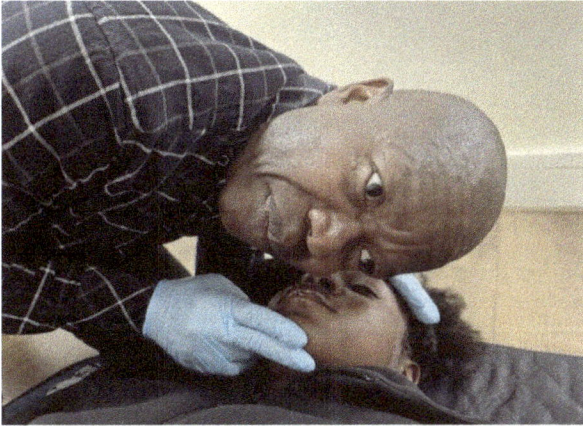

Reach for the casualty's hand nearest you and put it in an angled Or straight position.

Reach Out for The Casualty's Hand further from You. Place it On their Cheek And Hold It there.

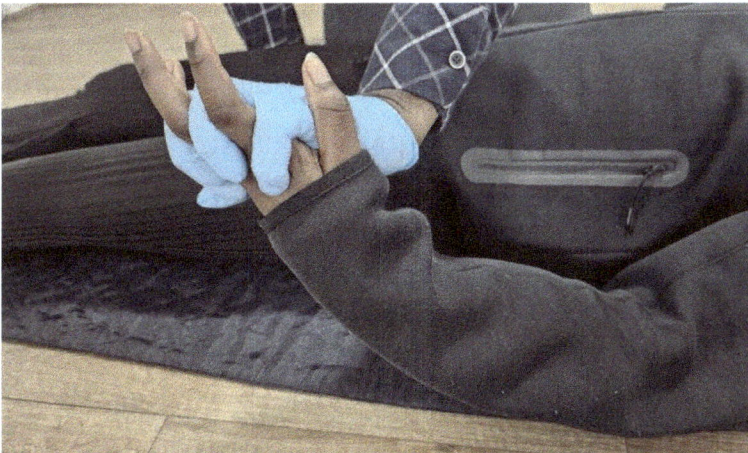

Place the back of the child's hand on their cheek and hold it palm to palm.

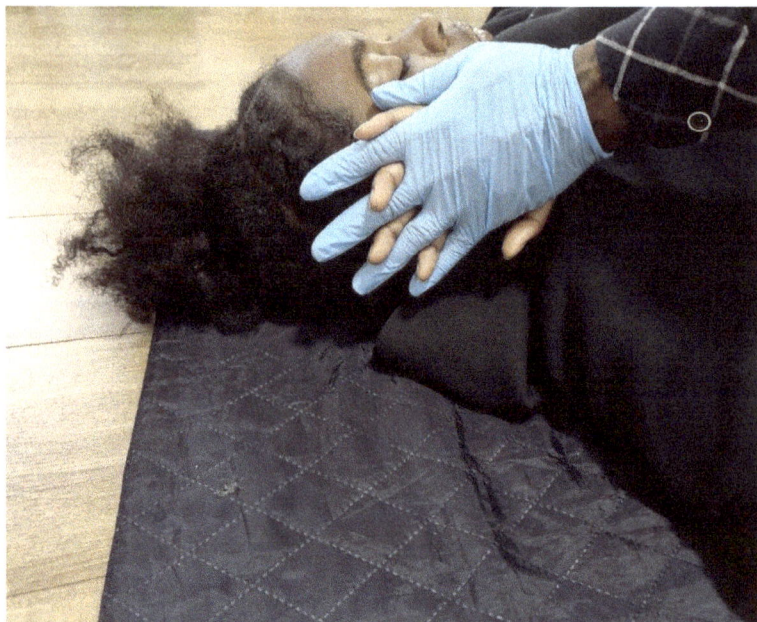

Check the pockets for any sharp objects likely to cause harm to the patient.

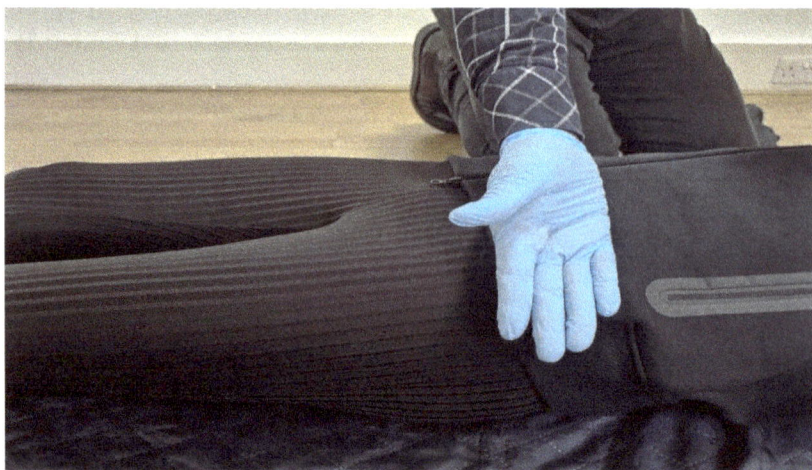

Check the pockets for Sharp objects that can harm the child when you are on her side.

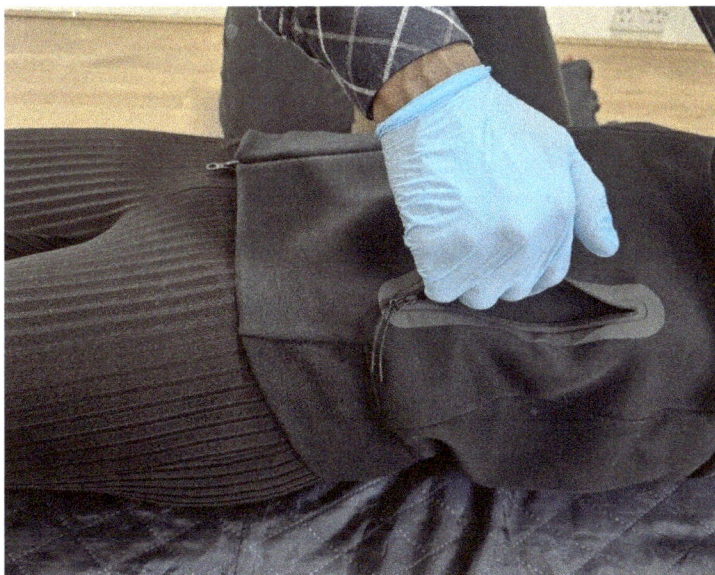

Place your hand on the outer part of the child's leg, which is furthest from you, around the knee.

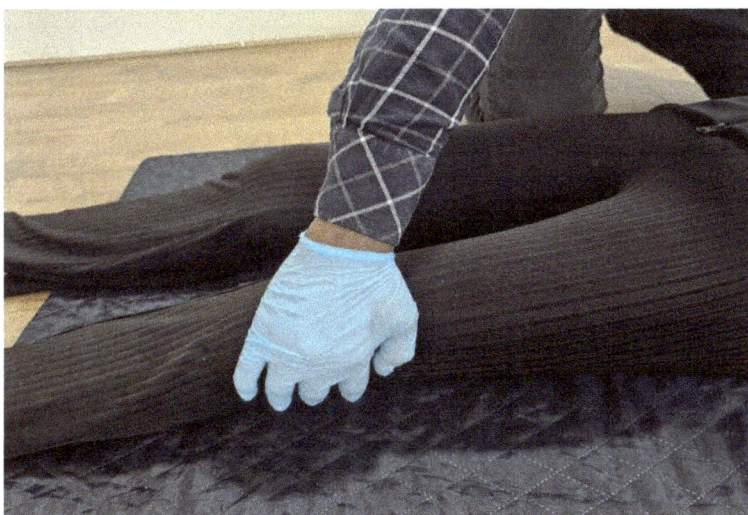

Reach for the leg farther from you and raise it from the Outer part of the knee area, Making Sure the feet are firmly on the ground. Then, lean the casualty towards you.

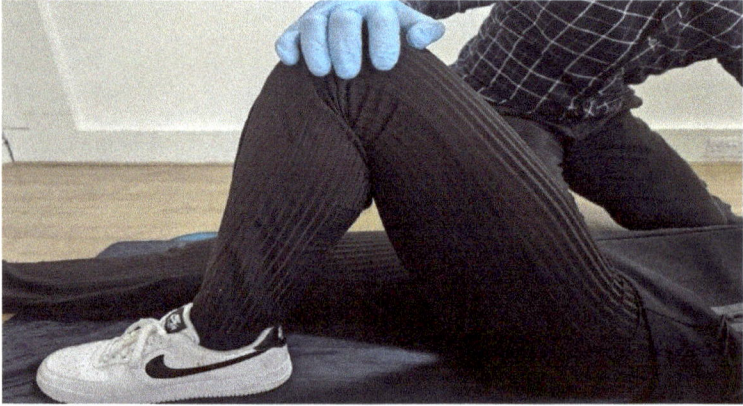

Lift the leg with your hand on the child's knee. Using the knee as a lever, roll the child on her side in a recovery position. Tilt the head back carefully to maintain a clear airway. Check every minute to confirm the child is still breathing whilst waiting for an ambulance to arrive.

TILT THE CHIN UP TO CLEAR THE CASUALTY'S AIRWAY

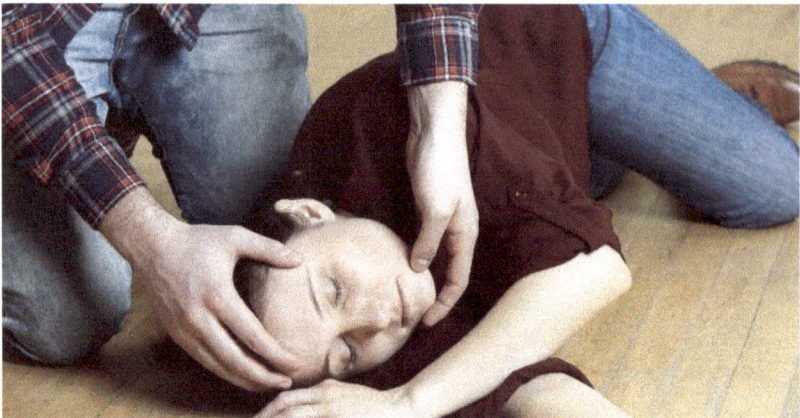

RECOVERY POSITION BABY

CHECK IF BABY IS RESPONSIVE

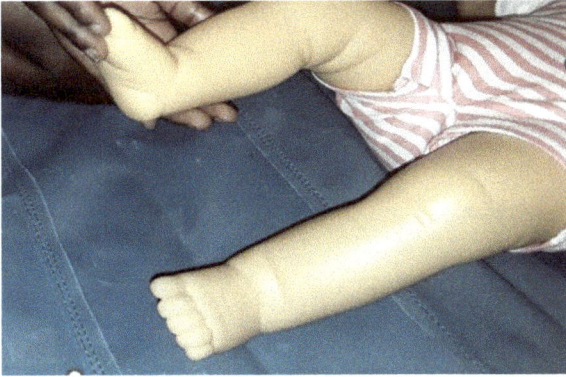

CALL 999/112 IF BABY IS UNRESPONSIVE

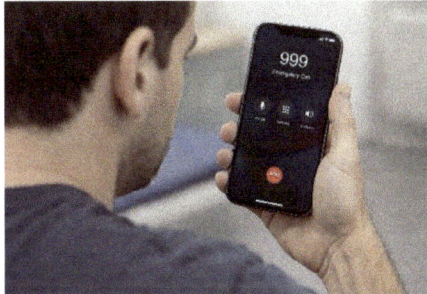

CHECK THE AIRWAY- HEAD TILT AND CHIN LIFT.

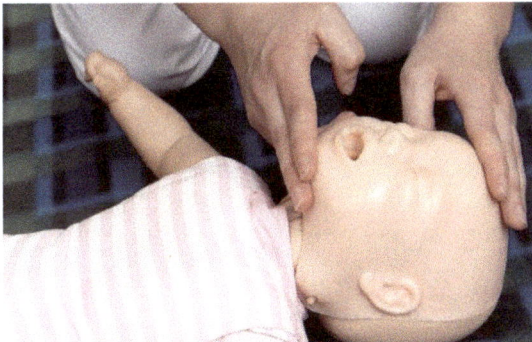

CHECK BREATHING.

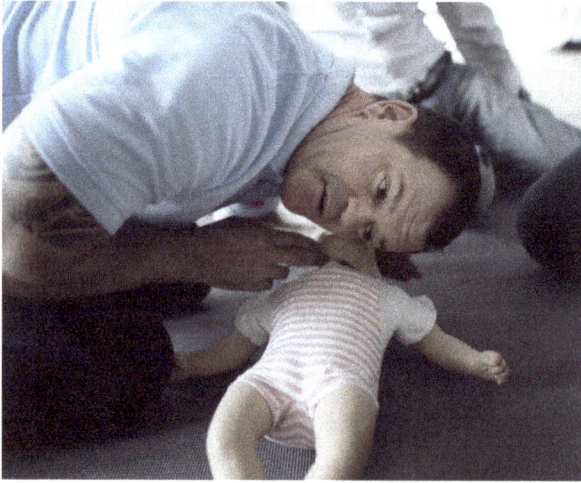

HOLD IN SIDE-LYING OR PRONE POSITION

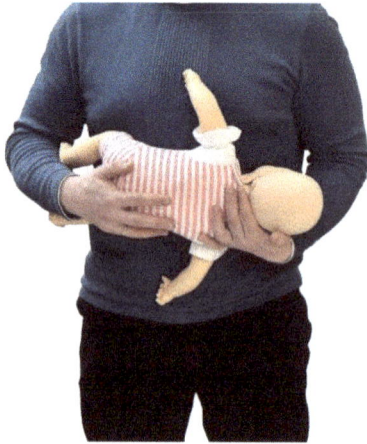

- Head lower than body
- Maintain airway alignment

USING THE AUTOMATED EXTERNAL DEFIBRILLATOR

ADULT CHOKING

WHAT IS CHOKING?

Choking occurs when the airway is partially or fully blocked, preventing air from reaching the lungs. This can happen anywhere from the mouth down to where the windpipe splits into the lungs.

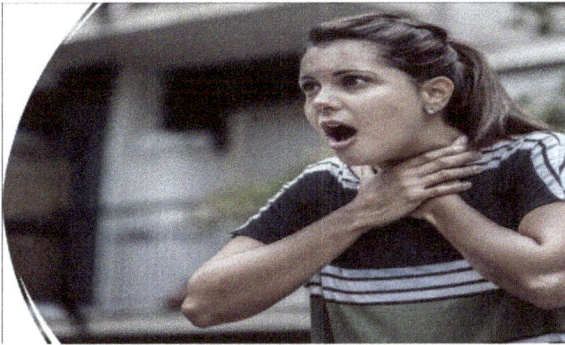

Mild Choking- adult

Mild choking occurs when the airway is only partially blocked, and the patient can still **breathe, cough, or speak**.

- **What to do:**
  - Encourage the patient to **cough forcefully**.
  - Do **not interfere** if they can clear the obstruction themselves.
  - **Do not give back blows or chest thrusts** unless the airway becomes entirely blocked.

Severe Choking

Severe choking usually involves complete blockage of the airway. The person will not be able to speak. To help them, you must immediately commence five back lows followed by five abdominal thrusts. If the treatment does not work, the patient will, at some point, become unconscious and not breathing. It would be best if you commenced CPR immediately.

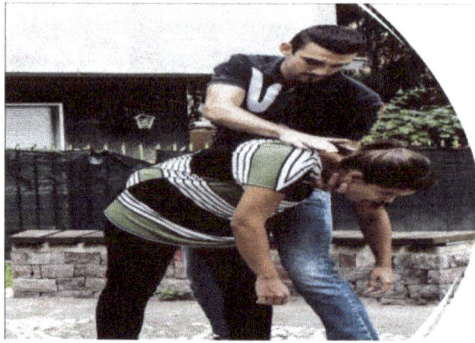

Abdominal thrusts

Make a fist with your dominant hand, and then place that fist above the navel and below the tip of the sternum. Press backward and upwards up to five times.

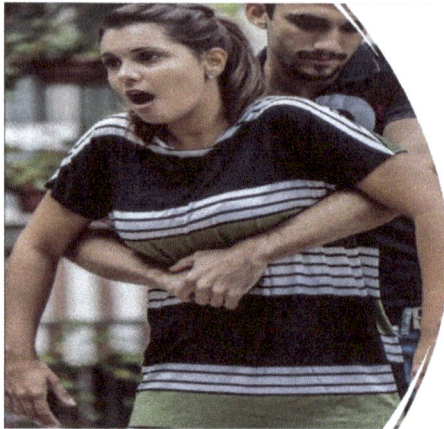

DENTAL PRACTICE CHOKING GUIDE

COMMON CAUSES IN PATIENTS

- Eating too quickly
- Loose or poorly fitting dentures
- Eating while lying down
- Not chewing properly
- Small objects, toys, or teeth
- Vomit

DENTAL INSTRUMENTS AND MATERIALS THAT CAN CAUSE CHOKING

- Root canal files
- Dental burs
- Cotton wool
- Water or saliva

Signs of a child choking

- Suspect a foreign-body airway obstruction if a child or adolescent cannot speak, breathe, or cough effectively.
- **Call 999 or 112**
- Call **for help** if the obstruction persists or the patient shows signs of severe choking.

EMERGENCY ACTIONS FOR INFANTS (<1 YEAR)

KEY POINTS FOR DENTAL TEAMS

- Always **stop treatment immediately** if a patient starts choking.
- Keep **airway clear of instruments, water, and saliva**.
- Ensure **oxygen and suction** are available in every clinical area.
- **AED should be immediately accessible**, including paediatric pads for children.
- Practice **regular training drills** for both adults and children.

How to help a choking child

Follow these steps if the child is choking:

1. CALL 999 FOR AN AMBULANCE

Ask for an ambulance and tell them the child is choking

My child is choking!

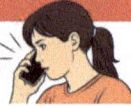

THEN

1. Give up to 5 back blows

Lean the child forward

Give 5 sharp back blows between the shoulder blades

Check if the choking is relieved after each blow

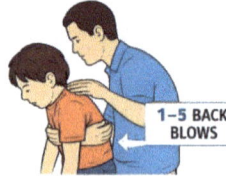

1–5 BACK BLOWS

2. Give up to 5 back blows:

If still choking, give abdominal thrusts:

Stand behind the child

Place your fist in the middle of the abdomen

Pull inwards and upwards up to 5 times

Check if the choking is relieved after each thrust

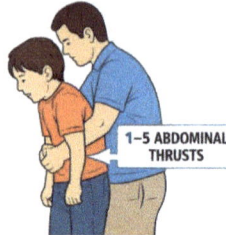

1–5 ABDOMINAL THRUSTS

✓ Continue with 5 back blows and 5 abdominal thrusts

✓ Follow the call handler's advice until help arrives

SIGNS OF A CHOKING INFANT

- Suspect choking due to a foreign object when an infant cries aloud (infants or more minor children) when feeding, eating, or playing unsupervised.

CALL FOR 999 OR 112

- Call or have someone call the ambulance service as soon as possible.

GIVE 5 BACK BLOWS

Position the infant face down along your forearm, resting your arm on your thigh. Support the head and keep it lower than the chest. Deliver up to five sharp back blows between the shoulder blades, checking after each blow to see if the obstruction has cleared.

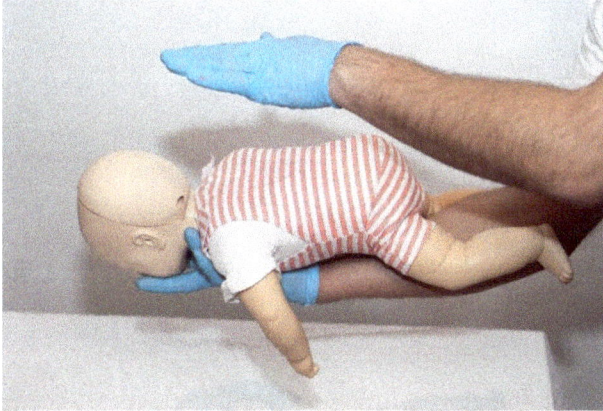

Chest Thrust with two thumbs encircling technique

Place the baby on their back on your lap. Wrap your hands around their chest and use your thumbs to give up to five quick pushes on the middle of the chest. Check after each push to see if the object has come out.

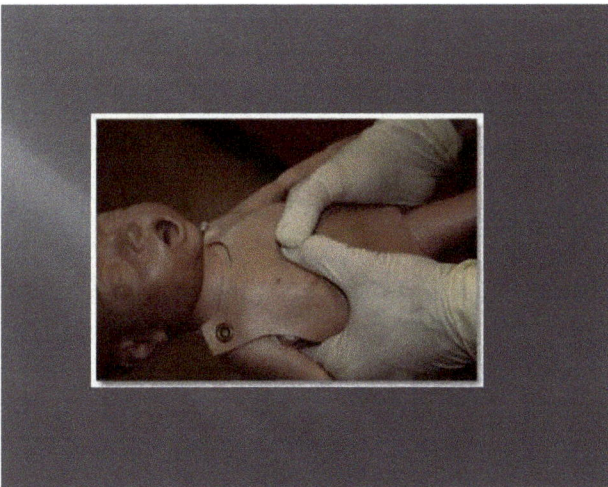

NO BLIND FINGER SWEEPS

Do not put your fingers blindly into the baby's mouth. Remove the object only if you can see it clearly.

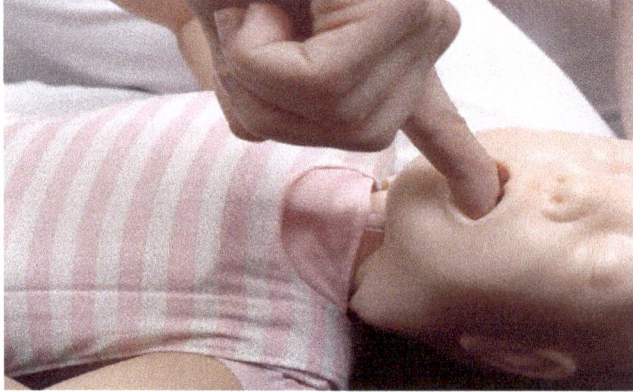

Do not put your fingers blindly into the baby's mouth. Remove the object only if you can see it clearly.

RESUSCITATION COUNCIL GUIDELINES ON THE USE OF SUCTION-BASED AIRWAY CLEARANCE DEVICES, SUCH AS LIFEVAC, FOR INDIVIDUALS CHOKING IN A DENTAL PRACTICE.

The Resuscitation Council does not yet support the use of these devices because:

a. There are insufficient evidence and research on the safety of these anti-choking devices.
b. There is no evidence that they are effective.
c. The use of the devices may delay the use of established treatments for choking.
d. Trained healthcare professionals already use advanced techniques such as suction, laryngoscopes, and forceps to remove foreign bodies stuck in the airway.

AUDITING RESUSCITATION EQUIPMENT (Dental & Clinical Settings)

- **Weekly equipment checks**
- Document findings
- Replace expired or faulty items
- Conduct **debriefs after any cardiac arrest**
- Take immediate corrective action

OXYGEN

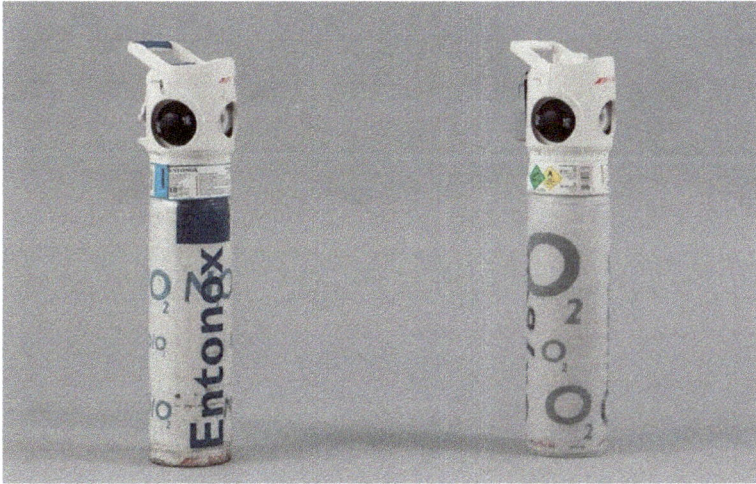

Oxygen Therapy in the Clinical Environment

Oxygen is a commonly used emergency drug in healthcare settings and must be administered **safely, appropriately, and according to national guidance**. In dental and primary care environments, the main gases encountered are **medical oxygen** and **Entonox® (50% oxygen / 50% nitrous oxide)**, both supplied in compressed cylinders of varying sizes.[31]

Types of Medical Gases

Medical Oxygen

- A **prescription-only medicine** used to treat hypoxaemia
- Delivered via masks or airway devices at controlled flow rates

Entonox®

- A fixed mixture of **50% oxygen and 50% nitrous oxide**
- Used primarily for **analgesia**, not routine oxygen therapy
- Requires specific training and equipment

Oxygen Equipment: Components

An emergency oxygen kit should include:

- Medical-grade oxygen cylinder
- Regulator with flow meter
- Oxygen tubing
- Non-rebreather mask with reservoir bag
- Bag-valve-mask (BVM) with reservoir
- Therapy (simple) face mask
- Resuscitation mask

Cylinders should be stored securely and handled in accordance with local safety policies.[32]

Oxygen Equipment Assembly (Emergency Use)

1. Place the oxygen cylinder securely (upright or safely supported)
2. Attach the **regulator** firmly to the cylinder
3. Connect oxygen tubing to the selected delivery device (mask or BVM)
4. Turn the cylinder **on slowly**
5. Set the flow rate according to clinical need

Flow Rate in Critical Illness

- **15 litres per minute (L/min)** via:
  - Non-rebreather mask
  - Bag-valve-mask with reservoir

6. Apply the mask securely over the patient's mouth and nose
7. Continuously monitor the patient's response and vital signs[33]

Discontinuing Oxygen Therapy

- Remove the oxygen mask when clinically appropriate
- Turn off the cylinder valve
- Allow the pressure gauge to fall to zero
- Disconnect equipment and replace the cylinder if empty

Record oxygen use in the patient chart.

Oxygen Delivery Devices

Non-Rebreather Mask

- Delivers **high-concentration oxygen**
- Flow rate: **10–15 L/min**
- Includes a reservoir bag and one-way valves to prevent re-breathing[33]

Simple Face Mask

- Has side ports allowing entrainment of room air
- Delivers **moderate oxygen concentrations**
- Requires flow rates ≥5 L/min to prevent CO_2 rebreathing

Venturi Mask

- Uses colour-coded valves to deliver **fixed oxygen concentrations**
- Particularly useful for patients at risk of **hypercapnic respiratory failure** (e.g. COPD)[34]

Nasal Cannula

- Delivers low-flow oxygen via nasal prongs
- Flow rate: **1–4 L/min**
- Suitable for stable patients with mild hypoxia

Nebuliser

- Used to deliver **aerosolised medications**, not oxygen alone
- Oxygen or air may be used as the driving gas depending on the indication

Oxygen: Clinical Classification

- **Drug class:** Medical gas
- **Action:** Increases oxygen availability for cellular metabolism
- **Indications include:**
  - Hypoxaemia
  - Cardiac arrest
  - Shock
  - Severe asthma
  - Anaphylaxis
  - Carbon monoxide poisoning
  - Major trauma[33]

Adverse Effects and Cautions

- Excessive oxygen may:
  - Reduce respiratory drive in patients with **chronic CO_2 retention**
  - Cause **hypercapnia** in susceptible individuals (e.g. COPD)
  - Lead to coronary vasoconstriction in certain cardiac conditions[34]

Oxygen should be **titrated to target saturations**, not given indiscriminately except in life-threatening emergencies.

Contraindications

- **Paraquat poisoning**
  Oxygen may worsen lung injury and should be avoided unless specifically advised by toxicology services[35]

Oxygen Dosage Summary (Adults)

Delivery Method	Flow Rate
Nasal cannula	1–4 L/min
Simple face mask	≥5 L/min
Venturi mask	As per valve colour
Non-rebreather mask	10–15 L/min
BVM with reservoir	15 L/min

References (continuing numbering)

31. British Thoracic Society. *Guideline for Oxygen Use in Adults in Healthcare and Emergency Settings*
32. Health and Safety Executive. *Safe Use of Compressed Gas Cylinders*
33. Resuscitation Council UK. *Emergency Oxygen Use and Adult Basic Life Support*
34. NICE. *Chronic Obstructive Pulmonary Disease in Over 16s (NG115)*
35. TOXBASE / UK National Poisons Information Service. *Paraquat Poisoning*

Anaphylaxis

Anaphylaxis is a **severe, rapid-onset, life-threatening allergic reaction** caused by the sudden release of mediators (like histamine) from mast cells and basophils. It can affect **multiple body systems** at once—especially the **airway, breathing, and circulation**—and requires **immediate emergency treatment**.

What happens in anaphylaxis

Anaphylaxis typically develops **within minutes** of exposure to an allergen and may include:

- **Airway:** throat tightness, swelling of tongue/lips, hoarseness, stridor
- **Breathing:** wheeze, shortness of breath, chest tightness
- **Circulation:** hypotension, dizziness, collapse, shock
- **Skin:** urticaria (hives), flushing, itching, angioedema
- **GI:** nausea, vomiting, abdominal cramps

Key point: Skin signs may be absent—do not rule out anaphylaxis if airway or circulatory symptoms are present.

Common causes of anaphylaxis in a dental practice

1. Local anaesthetics (rare, but important)

- True allergy is **rare**
- Reactions are more commonly due to:
  - **Preservatives** (e.g., sulphites)
  - **Latex contamination** of cartridges
- Ester-type LAs (rarely used) have a higher allergy risk than amide types

2. Antibiotics

- **Penicillin and cephalosporins** (most common)

- Can occur even if the patient has taken them before without problems

3. Latex

- Gloves, rubber dams, elastic bands
- Higher risk in:
    - Patients with multiple surgeries
    - Spina bifida
    - Healthcare workers
- Symptoms may worsen with repeated exposure during treatment

4. Chlorhexidine

- Found in:
    - Mouthwashes
    - Gels
    - Impregnated dressings
- Increasingly recognized cause of **peri-procedural anaphylaxis**

5. Analgesics

- **NSAIDs** (e.g., ibuprofen, aspirin)
- Can trigger anaphylaxis or severe bronchospasm in susceptible patients

6. Other potential triggers

- Acrylics, impression materials (rare)
- Flavouring agents or additives
- Topical antibiotics

Why this matters in dentistry

- Anaphylaxis is **unpredictable**

- Can occur **even without a known allergy**
- Dental teams must be prepared for **immediate recognition and management**, including:
  - Prompt use of **IM adrenaline (epinephrine)**
  - Calling emergency services
  - Airway and oxygen support

Dental Anaphylaxis Recognition Checklist

Suspect ANAPHYLAXIS if there is:

Sudden onset (minutes) after exposure *PLUS* **airway, breathing or circulation compromise**

Airway (A)

☐ Throat tightness
☐ Hoarse voice / difficulty speaking
☐ Swollen tongue, lips, or face
☐ Stridor

Breathing (B)

☐ Shortness of breath
☐ Wheeze / bronchospasm
☐ Rapid breathing
☐ Cyanosis
☐ SpO_2 falling

Circulation (C)

☐ Dizziness or collapse
☐ Hypotension
☐ Tachycardia

☐ Pale, clammy skin
☐ Loss of consciousness

Skin / Mucosa (may be absent)

☐ Urticaria (hives)
☐ Flushing
☐ Itching
☐ Angioedema

Dental Anaphylaxis Emergency Protocol

IMMEDIATE ACTIONS (ABCDE approach)

1. STOP treatment

- Remove allergen
- Lie the patient **flat** unless they are struggling to breathe while lying on their back
- If breathing difficulty, get them to sit in a **semi-reclined position**
- If pregnant, put the patient in a **left lateral tilt**

2. CALL FOR HELP

- Shout for assistance
- **Call 999or 112 immediately**

3. ADRENALINE (Epinephrine) – FIRST LINE OF TREATMENT

Do NOT delay

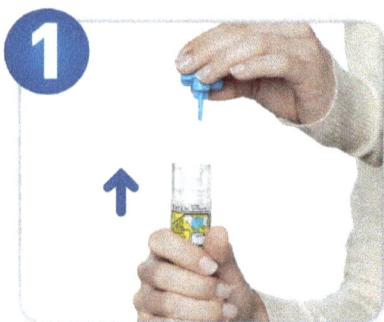

Form fist around EpiPen® and
BLUE SAFETY RELEASE

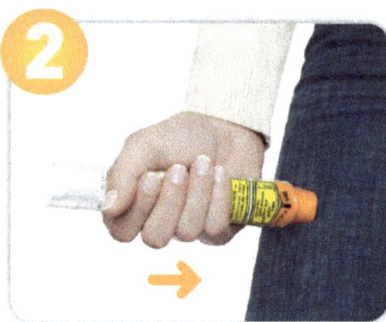

Push **ORANGE** end hard into outer
thigh so it 'clicks' and hold for 3 s‡

‡After administration of EpiPen® Adrenaline Auto-Injector
always seek medical attention – call **999 / 112**

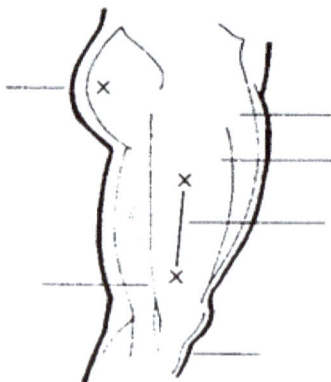

Route:

Intramuscular (IM)
Anterolateral thigh (vastus lateralis)

HOW TO USE THE EPIPEN

STEP 1

Form your fist around the EpiPen and remove the safety cap by pulling it straight up.

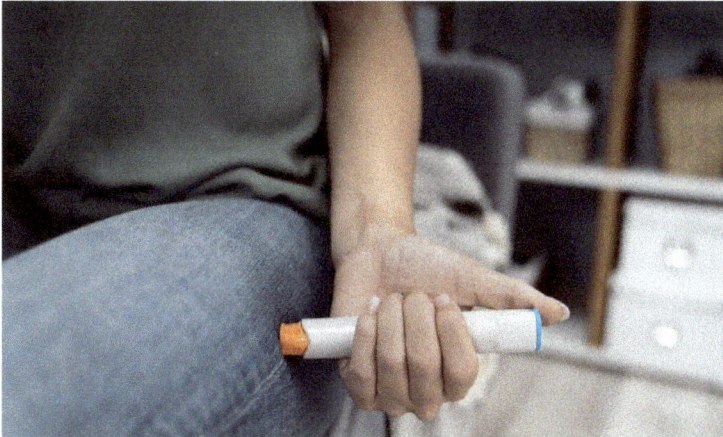

STEP 2

Swing and push the orange part of the auto-injector firmly against the anterolateral thigh until it "clicks." Hold the injection in place for 3 seconds. Count "1,2,3" slowly.

STEP 3

After injection, the orange cover automatically extends to ensure the needle is never exposed.

STEP 4

Isolate the casualty from the trigger.

Make sure the casualty is isolated from the trigger. Remove the stinger stuck to the skin if a bee has stung the casualty.

RECOMMENDED NEEDLE LENGTH

The Resuscitation Council recommends that the length be 25mm for all ages, based on a recommendation from Public Health England.[1]

Dental practice should have adrenaline 1:1000 (1mg/ml) ampoules in their emergency drugs kit. Anaphylaxis packs should have the following:

- Adrenaline 1:1000 ampoules x 2

- Blue 23G 25 mm needles x 4

- Graduated 1 ml syringes x 4.

Some dental practices prefer pre-filled syringes. The advantage of the pre-filled syringes is that they prevent the need to draw the medication from an ampoule.

The injection should be administered in the anterolateral aspect of the middle third of the thigh, but if that is not possible, it should be administered on the arm.

ADRENALINE AUTO INJECTOR OR AMPOULES-WHICH IS BETTER FOR TREATING ANAPHYLAXIS?

It is up to the individual clinical environment to determine whether to use the ampoule or an adrenaline auto-injector. The ampoules are cheaper, and their supply is more dependable as they are not prone to the supply chain issues that affect adrenaline auto-injectors. The needles are longer, and it is necessary to give the appropriate dose, especially for obese patients. In the heat of the moment, drawing the

---

[1] Public Health England. Immunisation against infectious disease. 2014. Available online
at https://www.gov.uk/government/collections/immunisation-against-infectious-disease-the-green-book (accessed April 2020).

right amounts of adrenaline from an ampoule with a syringe may be problematic. Errors are sometimes unavoidable.

Adrenaline auto-injectors are made for self-use by patients and are prescribed for each patient. They are expensive and have a limited shelf life. Most auto-injectors deliver 300 mcg of adrenaline to adults, less than the recommended dose for adults and teenagers, which is 500 mcg.

The needles for the standard auto-injectors are not long enough for some patients. For example, the EpiPen has a 16 mm needle to administer 300 mcg. The Resuscitation Council recommends that a standard blue needle (25mm and 23G) be used to inject intramuscular adrenaline. Still, a longer needle (38 mm in length and 21 G) may be needed for larger patients.

GRADUATED ADRENALINE, SYRINGE, AND NEEDLE

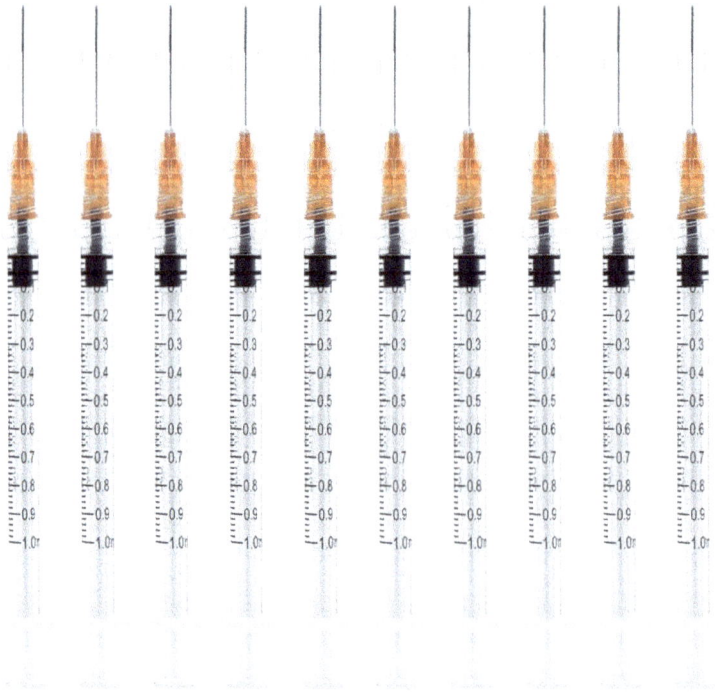

THE AMPOULE-1: 1000

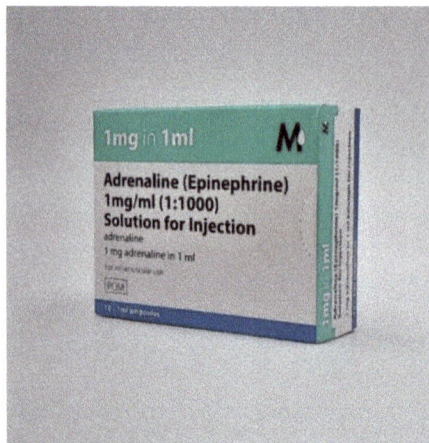

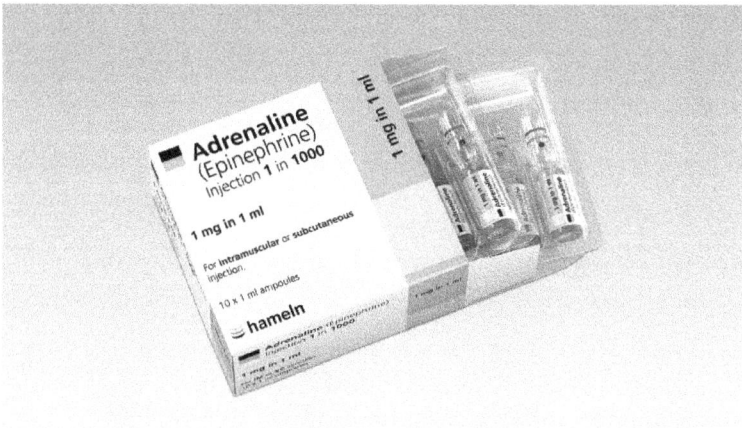

Adrenaline Dosing (IM)

Patient	Dose	Concentration
Adult	500 mcg	1:1000 (1 mg/mL)
Child 6–12 yrs	300 mcg	1:1000 (1 mg/mL)
Child >6mths-<6yrs	150 mcg	1:1000(1mg/mL)
Infant 0-6mths	100 mcg	1: 1000 (mg/mL)

Repeat every 5 minutes if no improvement.

4. AIRWAY & BREATHING SUPPORT

☐ High-flow **oxygen (15 L/min)** via mask
☐ Prepare suction
☐ Monitor SpO$_2$
☐ Be ready for airway obstruction

5. CIRCULATION

☐ Keep patient warm
☐ Monitor pulse & BP
☐ If trained and available → IV fluids

SECONDARY MEDICATIONS (Do NOT delay adrenaline)

(Given after adrenaline)

Antihistamines (e.g. chlorphenamine or cetirizine)

Antihistamines are **not indicated for the initial management of anaphylaxis** and **must not delay the administration of intramuscular adrenaline**, which remains the first-line treatment for life-threatening reactions.

They have **no benefit in treating airway, breathing, or circulatory compromise** and do not prevent or reverse shock. Their role is limited to the relief of **persistent cutaneous symptoms**, such as urticaria or pruritus.

Antihistamines should **only be administered once the patient is fully stabilised**, following appropriate emergency treatment. In this context, a **non-sedating oral antihistamine**, such as **cetirizine**, is preferred when the patient can safely swallow.

Routine administration of corticosteroids (e.g., hydrocortisone) is not advised, as there is no reliable evidence that it improves outcomes or prevents biphasic reactions.

Salbutamol for persistent bronchospasm. It must not be used instead of adrenaline, but can be administered where there is persistent bronchospasm despite administering adrenaline

OBSERVATION & HANDOVER

- Patient **must be transferred to the hospital**

- Risk of **biphasic reaction** (up to 24 hrs)
- Document:
    - Trigger
    - Time of onset
    - Drugs & doses
    - Response

Common Pitfalls in Dental Settings

- Delaying adrenaline
- Confusing anaphylaxis with vasovagal syncope
- Sitting patient upright with hypotension
- Relying on skin signs alone

WHO CAN ADMINISTER THE ADENALINE AMPOULES?

Legal Basis for Emergency Adrenaline Use

Under the **Prescription Only Medicines (Human Use) Order 1997**, certain injectable drugs (including **adrenaline for anaphylaxis**) *may be administered by anyone in a life-saving emergency* to save a life, even **without a prescription**. This includes adrenaline ampoules drawn up and given by syringe and needle.[2]

Who Can Administer Adrenaline Ampoules in a Dental Practice

1. Dentists

✓ **Always permitted** to administer adrenaline ampoules intramuscularly in a medical emergency
✓ Must be trained and competent in drawing up and administering IM injections

---

[2] psm.sdcep.org.uk

As registered clinicians, dentists have clinical autonomy and are responsible for providing emergency care, including intramuscular adrenaline for **anaphylaxis**.[3]

2. Dental Hygienists and Dental Therapists

✓ **Can administer adrenaline** IF:

- They are **competent and trained** in emergency management and IM injections
- They are working **within their scope of practice** and local protocols

The **GDC** references Resuscitation Council guidance, which forms the standard for emergency drugs and training. Hygienists/therapists may hold and use emergency drugs on site, but must have appropriate training and protocols in place. (General Dental Council)

Note: Direct drug supply/administration rules are evolving, but in emergencies the *Prescription Only Medicines (Human Use) Order* allows life-saving use irrespective of prescription status. (psm.sdcep.org.uk)

3. Dental Nurses and Other Team Members

✓ **May administer adrenaline ampoules** *in a life-saving emergency* if:

- They are **trained and competent** in emergency procedures
- They act under the **practice's medical emergency protocol and supervision**
- The situation is **a genuine anaphylactic emergency**

---

[3] General Dental Council

Resuscitation Council UK and SDCEP both make it clear that *anyone present who is competent* can administer adrenaline in anaphylaxis to save a life. (psm.sdcep.org.uk)

Important Clarifications

Training & Competence

All team members who **might administer adrenaline ampoules** must be:

- **Trained** in medical emergencies, including anaphylaxis recognition and IM injection
- **Practised regularly** with mock scenarios
- Up-to-date with resuscitation skills as expected by the Resuscitation Council and GDC standards (General Dental Council)

The GDC states that *every registrant must know their role in a medical emergency and be sufficiently trained and competent to carry out that role*. (cpd4dentalnurses.co.uk)

*The Prescription Only Medicines (Human Use) Order 1997 [1] lists injectable drugs that can be administered by anyone for the purpose of saving a life in an emergency; this includes adrenaline and glucagon. Therefore, all dental team members may administer adrenaline and glucagon, and the non-injectable drugs listed below. However, dental team members must be competent in the use of these drugs, and employers must accept responsibility for the actions of staff." (SDCEP-The Scottish Dental SDCEP Clinical effectiveness Programme)

- Examples of the injectable drugs listed are Adrenaline, 1 ml ampoules or pre-filled syringes of 1:1000 solution for intramuscular injection.
- Glucagon, for intramuscular injection of 1 mg.

"Dental practices might wish to stock the following to aid the management of patients with mild allergic reactions

- Cetirizine, 10 mg tablets, or oral solution (5 mg/5 ml).
- Chlorphenamine, 4 mg tablets or oral solution (2 mg/5 ml); (NB: chlorphenamine can cause drowsiness)

Loratadine, 10 mg tablets or syrup (5 mg/5 ml)." (SDCEP-The Scottish Dental Clinical Effectiveness Programme)

Human Medicines Regulations 2012

Use of Intramuscular Adrenaline by Anyone

◆ The Key Legal Provision

The relevant part of the Human Medicines Regulations 2012 is
Regulation 238
(*Exemptions for the administration of prescription-only medicines in an emergency*).

What the Law Explicitly Allows

Regulation 238 permits:

Any person to administer a **Prescription Only Medicine (POM)**
by injection
for the purpose of saving life
in an emergency

This exemption applies **even if**:

- The person is **not a prescriber**
- The medicine is normally **prescription-only**
- There is **no Patient Specific Direction (PSD)** or **Patient Group Direction (PGD)**

How This Applies to Adrenaline

- **Adrenaline (epinephrine)** is a **Prescription Only Medicine**
- IM adrenaline is the **first-line treatment for anaphylaxis**

- Anaphylaxis is a **life-threatening emergency**

Therefore, **any person** may legally administer **IM adrenaline** in an emergency **to save life**, provided the situation is genuine.

Application in a Dental Practice

Under **HMR 2012 Regulation 238**:

The following may administer IM adrenaline in anaphylaxis:

- Dentists
- Dental hygienists
- Dental therapists
- Dental nurses
- Any other trained person present

✓ **No prescription required**
✓ **No PGD required**
✓ **No professional registration required**

The legal authority comes **directly from the Regulations**, not from professional scope alone.

Important Conditions and Safeguards

Although legally permitted, the following still apply:

1 **Emergency Only**

- Must be a **life-threatening situation**
- Routine or precautionary use is **not covered**

2 **Route Matters**

- IM adrenaline is appropriate
- **IV adrenaline is NOT covered** and is unsafe in primary care

③ Professional Accountability

- GDC standards still apply:
  - Act within competence
  - Be trained
  - Be able to justify actions

The exemption allows administration, **not poor practice**.

Alignment with National Guidance

Resuscitation Council (UK)

- Explicitly supports **IM adrenaline by trained responders**
- Emphasises **do not delay adrenaline**

NICE / BNF

- Recognises adrenaline as **first-line** for anaphylaxis
- Notes emergency use without prescription

GDC

- Requires registrants to:
  - Know their role in emergencies
  - Be trained and competent
  - Act in patients' best interests

HMR 2012 provides the **legal permission**; professional bodies provide the **practice standards**.

Summary Table

Team Member	Can administer adrenaline ampoule?	Conditions
Dentist	Yes	Always, with training

Team Member	Can administer adrenaline ampoule?	Conditions
Hygienist / Therapist	Yes	With training + within scope + protocols
Dental Nurse / Other	Yes	In a true emergency with competency & practice protocol
Clinical Dental Technician	Not expected to hold/administer emergency kit medicines	GDC does *not* expect CDTs to have emergency drug kits[4] (General Dental Council)

CQC / GDC Compliance Checklist – Medical Emergencies & Adrenaline Use

Practice Name: _____   Date of Audit: _____

Governance & Policies	
Written medical emergencies policy in place	■
Policy includes anaphylaxis & adrenaline ampoules	■
Policy reviewed annually	■

Emergency Drugs & Equipment	
Adrenaline 1:1000 ampoules available and in-date	■
Syringes & IM needles available	■
Oxygen with masks and tubing available	■
Emergency drugs checked regularly	■

Training & Competence	
All clinical staff trained annually	■
Training includes IM adrenaline administration	■
Emergency drills carried out	■

Documentation & Review	
Emergency incidents documented	■
Significant events reviewed and learning shared	■

Audit completed by: _____   Signature: _____

---

[4] General Dental Council

NASAL ADRENALINE SPRAY FOR ANAPHYLAXIS

What is EURneffy®?

EURneffy® is a **needle-free adrenaline (epinephrine) nasal spray** used for the **emergency treatment of severe allergic reactions (anaphylaxis)**. It offers an alternative to traditional adrenaline auto-injectors (AAIs). [5]

Why it matters:

Fast administration of adrenaline during anaphylaxis saves lives. A nasal spray may reduce hesitation to treat because it **avoids needles** and can be **used[6] quickly** in emergencies.

Regulatory Status

- GB **Approved by the UK's MHRA (July 2025)** — first needle-free option for anaphylaxis in the UK for adults and children ≥ 30 kg. Expected to be **available now (late 2025)**. (
- EU **Approved by the European Commission (2024)** — authorised across EU Member States.

Who Can Use It?

Adults and **children weighing 30 kg or more**
 Prescription-only medicine — must be prescribed by a healthcare professional. [7]

_____

[5] GOV.UK

[7] Anaphylaxis Campaign

How It Works (Quick Summary)

- A **single-use nasal spray** containing **2 mg adrenaline**.[8]
- Delivered **into one nostril only** — ready to use with no priming needed. (EURneffy®)
- Adrenaline is absorbed through the nasal lining and enters the bloodstream quickly to counteract anaphylaxis.[9]

When to Use It

Use EURneffy **as soon as signs of anaphylaxis appear**, such as:

- Difficulty breathing or wheeze
- Throat tightness or swelling
- Light-headedness/collapse
- Rapid onset of hives and low blood pressure

Administer immediately and call 999 — adrenaline is time-critical in anaphylaxis. [10]

Important Dosing & Administration Notes

✓ **One dose per device.** After use, the device must be discarded. [11]

✓ **Carry two devices** at all times — a second dose may be needed if symptoms continue or worsen.[12]

✓ **Seek urgent medical help after use**, even if symptoms improve[13]

---

[8] EURneffy®
[9] Anaphylaxis Campaign
[10] European Medicines Agency (EMA)
[11] EURneffy®
[12] (Anaphylaxis Campaign)
[13](European Medicines Agency (EMA)

Compared to Auto-Injectors

Advantages

- **Needle-free** — easier use for some patients
- **Smaller and lighter** to carry
- **Better temperature stability** and potentially longer shelf life than some auto-injectors [14]

Note: Traditional auto-injectors remain widely used and established; Eureffy is an additional option. Proper training in all adrenaline delivery methods is still essential.

Safety & Side Effects

Common reported effects may include:

- Nasal discomfort or irritation
- Headache or congestion
- Throat irritation
- Nervousness, dizziness
  (*Common side effects seen with nasal adrenaline sprays in general — see full prescribing info for details.*) [15]

Key Learner Takeaways

- EURneffy is a **needle-free adrenaline spray** for emergency anaphylaxis treatment.
- Approved in the **UK and EU** for adults and children ≥ 30 kg.
- **Use immediately** on the first signs of anaphylaxis and **call emergency services**.

---

[14] (Pharma Focus Europe)

- Always **carry two devices**.
- Does **not replace emergency medical care** — hospital assessment is needed after use.

How to Use
EURneffy® Nasal Adrenaline Spray

Emergency treatment of severe allergic reaction (anaphylaxis)

1. CALL 999 IMMEDIATELY

2. REMOVE SAFETY CAP — PULL OFF

3. INSERT INTO 1 NOSTRIL

3. INSERT INTO 1 NOSTRIL — TILT HEAD BACK

USE ONE SPRAY ONLY | THEN SEEK MEDICAL HELP.

Use of Adrenaline Auto-Injectors Prescribed for a Named Patient

Is it permissible to administer an adrenaline auto-injector prescribed for one individual to a different patient?

No.
Under current UK medicines legislation, an **adrenaline auto-injector (AAI) that has been prescribed for a named individual may only be administered to that named person.**

Although **anyone may administer adrenaline to save a life in an emergency**, this legal exemption **does not extend to using a Prescription Only Medicine that has been specifically prescribed to someone else** when that medicine is an **adrenaline auto-injector**.

Legal Position (Summary)

- **Adrenaline (epinephrine)** is a Prescription Only Medicine (POM).
- **Human Medicines Regulations 2012 (Regulation 238)** allow *any person* to administer a POM **by injection** in a life-threatening emergency **to save life**.
- However, this exemption **does not permit the use of a patient-specific prescribed medicine on another person** when that medicine is an **adrenaline auto-injector**.

Resuscitation Council (UK) Statement

"Currently, the law does not allow a non-prescriber to administer an adrenaline auto-injector which has been specifically prescribed for a named person to someone other than the person for whom it has been prescribed."
— Resuscitation Council (UK)

This position is consistently reflected in national dental and medical emergency guidance.

Practical Examples in a Dental Practice

Permitted

- Any trained person may administer:
  - **Practice-owned adrenaline auto-injector**, or
  - **Practice-owned adrenaline ampoule (1:1000) IM**
- A patient's **own prescribed auto-injector** may be used **on that same patient**.

Not Permitted

- Using **Patient B's prescribed adrenaline auto-injector** to treat **Patient A**, even in an emergency.

Example Scenario

- Patient A develops anaphylaxis during dental treatment.
- Patient B (in the waiting room) has a prescribed adrenaline auto-injector.

Unlawful: Using Patient B's auto-injector on Patient A
Lawful:

- Using the **practice's emergency adrenaline auto-injector**, or
- Drawing up and administering **IM adrenaline from a practice-held ampoule**

Key Compliance Message for Practices

Dental practices must:

- Stock **practice-owned adrenaline auto-injectors and/or adrenaline ampoules**
- Ensure staff are trained to:
  - Recognise anaphylaxis
  - Administer IM adrenaline promptly

- Avoid reliance on **patient-specific prescribed medicines for other patients**

HYPERVENTILATION (Acute over-breathing / anxiety-related breathlessness)

What it is

Hyperventilation is **breathing faster and/or deeper than the body's metabolic needs** (often triggered by **panic, anxiety, pain, or fear**). This can lead to **excessive "blowing off" of carbon dioxide, which may cause light-headedness, tingling, and carpopedal spasm (cramping in the hands/feet**).

In respiratory guidance, this often sits within **disordered breathing/hyperventilation syndrome**, where symptoms can **mimic asthma** and other cardiopulmonary problems—so assessment matters.[16]

17

Signs and symptoms (common)

- Feeling unable to "get a deep breath"
- **Dizziness / light-headedness**
- **Tingling or numbness** (around mouth, fingers)
- **Palpitations**
- Chest tightness or chest pain (often non-cardiac, but treat cautiously)
- **Dry mouth**
- Trembling, sweating
- **Carpopedal spasm** (spasms/cramps in hands/feet)
- Anxiety, fear, tearfulness

---

[16] British Thoracic Society
[17] . (British Thoracic Society

Management in a dental practice

1) First: assess for serious causes (do not assume anxiety)

Use an **ABCDE approach** and check **vital signs** (respiratory rate, pulse, BP, temperature, level of consciousness, oxygen saturation if available). The NICE CKS on breathlessness emphasises an initial ABC assessment and deciding whether emergency admission is needed[18].

Red flags → call 999/112 (treat as an emergency until proven otherwise):

- Low SpO_2, cyanosis, severe wheeze/stridor
- Hypotension, collapse, altered consciousness
- Signs of anaphylaxis, severe asthma, chest pain suggestive of cardiac cause

2) Reassure and coach breathing (main treatment)

- Stop treatment, sit the patient **upright** and encourage relaxation.
- Use **calm reassurance** ("This is frightening but it will pass; I'll coach your breathing.")
- Coach **slow, controlled breathing**, for example:
  - **Pursed-lip breathing** (inhale gently through nose, exhale slowly through pursed lips)
  - Encourage slower rate and smaller breaths (avoid deep "gulping" breaths)

Breathing retraining that focuses on **reducing respiratory rate and/or tidal volume** is recommended as **first-line** for hyperventilation syndrome/disordered breathing.[19]

---

[18] CKS
[19] . (British Thoracic Society

✓ You can also use a simple cadence:
"In…2…3… Out…2…3…4…5" (longer out-breath)

3) Oxygen: only if indicated

Do **not** give oxygen routinely for simple hyperventilation if oxygen saturations are normal. BTS guidance stresses oxygen should be used appropriately and targeted to need (i.e., treat hypoxaemia rather than anxiety symptoms). (British Thoracic Society)

4) Avoid paper-bag rebreathing

Do **not** use paper-bag breathing in clinical settings: it risks worsening unrecognised **hypoxia** or other serious conditions presenting as "hyperventilation." (This is widely reflected in modern emergency care teaching; in dentistry, focus on assessment + coached breathing rather than rebreathing.)

SYNCOPE

Fainting is a brief loss of consciousness triggered by a temporary reduction of blood to the brain.

Vasovagal syncope (fainting) is a brief loss of consciousness typically triggered by a temporary reduction of blood flow to the brain.

Causes

Fainting occurs when there is a temporary reduction of blood and glucose in the brain due to a drop in cerebral blood pressure.

· It would Usually happen when the person is upright, soon after standing up

· It can happen when sitting down over prolonged periods of inactivity, and fainting can also be caused by

- -Drugs
- -Dehydration
- -Alcohol
- Loss of bodily fluid such as vomiting, bleeding, or diarrhoea.

Signs and symptoms

- Dizziness
- Sweating
- Blurred vision

Distortion of hearing before collapse

·Might involve jerking, which can stop in about twenty seconds

WHEN DOES IT STOP?

When the patient is in a supine position, the recovery is rapid. Raise both legs. Ensure they do not stand up too quickly after recovering. This is to give the blood pressure and heart time to stabilise.

Cardiac Syncope: Cardiac syncope results from cardiac dysrhythmia (tachycardia and bradycardia). This is not as common as vasovagal syncope. It can happen whilst the patient is at rest and during exercise.

Pre-existing heart disease is a risk factor.

Signs

- Impairment of consciousness lasting over a minute
- Not likely to cause convulsive movements of more than 20 seconds

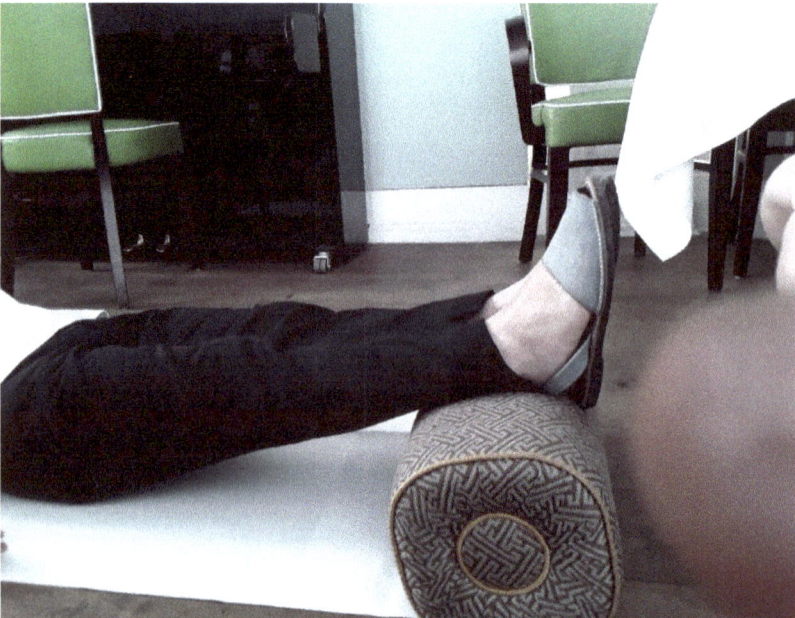

Adrenal Insufficiency

Adrenal insufficiency is a condition in which the adrenal glands fail to produce adequate cortisol and, sometimes, **aldosterone**, resulting in an inability to mount a normal stress response.

Types of Adrenal Insufficiency

Primary – Addison's disease

- The **adrenal glands themselves are damaged**
- They **cannot make enough cortisol**
- Lifelong condition
- Higher risk of **adrenal crisis**

Secondary / Tertiary – Steroid-related

- Caused by **long-term oral steroid use** (e.g. prednisolone)
- Steroids **switch off the body's normal cortisol system**
- The **HPA axis** (brain → adrenal signal pathway) becomes suppressed
- Risk can continue **months or years after stopping steroids**

Easy memory tip

- **Primary = gland problem (Addison's)**
- **Secondary/tertiary = steroid problem**

2 Why It Matters in Dentistry

- Dental treatment can cause **physiological stress** (pain, anxiety, infection)
- Patients with adrenal insufficiency **cannot increase cortisol production**
- This may lead to **adrenal crisis**, a **life-threatening emergency**

3 Causes Relevant to Dental Patients

- Addison's disease
- Long-term oral corticosteroid use (e.g. prednisolone)
- Recent cessation of long-term steroid therapy (risk persists for months to years)

4 Adrenal Crisis (Acute Adrenal Insufficiency)

Triggers

- Surgery or trauma
- Infection
- Severe pain or anxiety
- Vomiting / missed steroid doses
- Significant dental procedures in susceptible patients

Signs and Symptoms

- **Hypotension**
- Collapse/shock
- Severe weakness
- Nausea, vomiting
- Confusion or reduced consciousness
- Seizures
- Cardiac arrest (late)

Can be mistaken for syncope or sepsis — **think adrenal crisis in steroid-dependent patients**.

5 Steroid Cover – Current Guidance (Very Important)

Outdated Guidance:

"All dental procedures require steroid supplementation"

Current guidance:

Routine steroid supplementation is NOT required for most dental procedures, provided the patient continues their usual steroid dose.

Minor Dental Procedures

(e.g. scale and polish, simple fillings, routine LA)

- **No additional steroids required**
- Patient continues **normal daily dose**
- Reduce stress and ensure good LA

More Invasive Procedures

(e.g. surgical extraction, implants, prolonged procedures)

- **Individual risk assessment**
- Some patients may follow **"sick-day rules"**:
    - Double the usual oral steroid dose on the day
- Liaise with GP/endocrinologist **if unsure**

6 Practical Tips

✓ Morning appointments
✓ Short, well-planned visits
✓ Excellent pain control
✓ Avoid sudden cessation of steroids
✓ Ask patients to bring:

- **Steroid emergency card**
- **Hydrocortisone injection kit**
- **Adrenal crisis letter**

7 Adrenal Crisis in the Dental Chair

Immediate Management

1 **Stop treatment**
2 **Call 999 / 112**

→ say **"suspected Addisonian crisis"**
③ **Lay patient flat**, legs elevated
④ **Give high-flow oxygen**
⑤ **Administer IM hydrocortisone** (if available)
⑥ **Urgent transfer to the hospital**

⑧ **Emergency Hydrocortisone Doses (IM)**

Yes. In UK clinical practice, **hydrocortisone emergency doses are often expressed in both milligrams (mg) and millilitres (mL)**, based on the **standard UK emergency preparation**.

(Hydrocortisone sodium succinate 100 mg vial)

- Reconstituted with **2 mL** diluent
  → **Concentration = 50 mg/mL**

This is the preparation most supplied in:

- Emergency kits
- Addison's emergency injection kits
- NHS settings

Dose expressed in mg AND mL

Patient	Dose (mg)	Volume (mL)
Adult	100 mg IM	2 mL IM
Child ≥6 years	50–100 mg IM	1–2 mL IM
Infant (<1 year)	25 mg IM	0.5 mL IM

Think "100 mg = 2 mL"
→ Half the dose = half the volume

⑨ *Patients with adrenal insufficiency are at risk of adrenal crisis during physiological stress. Current guidance states that routine steroid supplementation is not required for most dental procedures if the patient continues their usual dose; however, adrenal crisis is a medical emergency treated with IM hydrocortisone, oxygen, and urgent hospital transfer.*

Diabetic Emergency Medication

Management of Hypoglycaemia

Hypoglycaemia is a **medical emergency** defined as a blood glucose level **<4.0 mmol/L**. Prompt recognition and treatment are essential to prevent neurological injury and loss of consciousness.[36]

Initial Management: Fast-Acting Carbohydrate (Conscious Patient)

Oral Glucose Administration

Indication:

- Conscious patient
- Able to swallow safely

Equipment Required:

- Gloves
- PPE
- Glucose preparation (oral liquid, tablets, gel, or sugar solution)

Procedure:

1. Explain the treatment and obtain verbal consent
2. Confirm the patient is conscious and able to swallow
3. Administer fast-acting carbohydrate orally or buccally
4. Recheck blood glucose after **10–15 minutes**
5. Repeat treatment if blood glucose remains <4.0 mmol/L
6. Once recovered, give **long-acting carbohydrate** to prevent recurrence[37]

Oral Glucose Options (Fast-Acting)

Option	Approximate Dose
Lift® / Glucojuice®	60–80 mL
Glucose tablets	4–5 tablets
Glucose 40% gel	1.5–2 tubes
Sugar dissolved in water	3–4 heaped teaspoons

Glucose 40% Oral Gel (Buccal Use)

Indications:

- Conscious but **uncooperative** patient
- Young children unable to drink

Administration:

- Apply gel **between the cheek and gum**
- Massage externally to aid absorption
- **Do NOT give to unconscious patients**

⚠ Aspiration risk:

If consciousness is reduced, oral glucose must **not** be administered[36].

Hypoglycaemia: Children (Age-Specific Management)

Children Aged 0–5 Years

Glucose 40% Oral Gel

- Administer **buccally only**
- Repeat after **10–15 minutes** if needed
- Measure blood glucose after each dose

Children Aged 5–11 Years

Route	Dose	Repeat
Oral	10 g glucose	
OR 40 mL Lift®		
OR 3 glucose tablets		
OR 1 tube glucose 40% gel		
OR 2 tsp sugar in water	After 15 minutes	
Buccal (uncooperative)	1 tube glucose 40% gel	After 15 minutes

Children Aged 12–17 Years

Route	Dose	Repeat
Oral	15 g glucose	
OR 60 mL Lift®		
OR 4 glucose tablets		
OR 1.5 tubes glucose 40% gel		
OR 3 tsp sugar in water	After 15 minutes	
Buccal (uncooperative)	15 g glucose	
OR 1.5 tubes glucose 40% gel		
OR 150–200 mL fruit juice	After 15 minutes	

Hypoglycaemia: Adults

Route	Dose	Repeat
Oral	15–20 g glucose	
OR 60–80 mL Lift®		
OR 4–5 glucose tablets		
OR 1.5–2 tubes glucose 40% gel		
OR 3–4 tsp sugar in water	After 15 minutes	
Buccal (uncooperative)	15–20 g glucose	

Route	Dose	Repeat
OR 1.5–2 tubes glucose 40% gel	After 15 minutes	

When Oral Treatment Is NOT Possible

Glucagon Injection (GlucaGen® 1 mg/mL)

Indication:

- Unconscious or fitting patient
- Blood glucose <4.0 mmol/L
- Oral glucose unsafe or impossible[38]

Mechanism of Action:

- Stimulates hepatic glycogen breakdown, increasing blood glucose

Important limitations:

- Less effective in:
    - Alcohol-related hypoglycaemia
    - Prolonged fasting
    - Liver disease
- Always follow with oral carbohydrate once conscious[38]

Glucagon Dosage (Intramuscular Only)

Age	Dose	Body Weight
0–8 years	500 micrograms (0.5 mL)	<25 kg
9–17 years	1 mg (1 mL)	≥25 kg
Adult	1 mg (1 mL)	—

Glucagon – Side Effects & Cautions

Side effects:

- Nausea and vomiting (common)
- Abdominal pain
- Hypotension
- Hypokalaemia (rare)
- Hypersensitivity reactions (very rare)

Cautions:

- Avoid repeat dosing if liver glycogen stores are depleted
- If ineffective, proceed to **IV glucose**[38]

Persistent Unresponsiveness After 10 Minutes

Intravenous Glucose (Advanced Care)

Medication	Age	Dose	Administration
Glucose 10%	Child	5 mL/kg (500 mg/kg)	IV via large vein
Glucose 10%	Adult	120–150 mL	IV over 15 minutes
Glucose 20%	Adult	75–100 mL	IV over 15 minutes

⚠ IV glucose administration requires **advanced clinical competence** and is not routinely delivered in dental practices.

Key Clinical Points for Dental Practice

- Hypoglycaemia = **blood glucose <4.0 mmol/L**
- **Never give oral glucose to an unconscious patient**
- Glucagon is a **temporary measure**
- Always give long-acting carbohydrate once recovered
- Call **999** if the patient does not respond or deteriorates[36]

References (continuing numbering)

36. Joint British Diabetes Societies (JBDS). *The Hospital Management of Hypoglycaemia*
37. NICE. *Diabetes in Adults and Children (NG17, NG18)*
38. Resuscitation Council UK. *Medical Emergencies in Primary Care and Dental Practice*

Septic Shock

(Sepsis With Circulatory Failure)

What Is Sepsis?

Sepsis is a **life-threatening organ dysfunction** caused by a **dysregulated host response to infection.**[39]
It is not the infection alone, but the body's abnormal immune response that leads to systemic inflammation, tissue injury, and organ failure.

What Is Septic Shock?

Septic shock is the **most severe form of sepsis** and is characterised by:[40]

- **Persistent hypotension** requiring urgent escalation
- **Evidence of inadequate tissue perfusion**
- Failure to respond adequately to initial fluid resuscitation (hospital setting)

Septic shock carries a **high mortality rate** and requires immediate hospital-level care.

Pathophysiology (Simplified)

- Infection triggers an exaggerated inflammatory response
- Release of inflammatory mediators causes:
  - Widespread **vasodilation**
  - **Increased capillary permeability**
- This results in:
  - Relative hypovolaemia
  - Reduced tissue perfusion
  - Progressive organ dysfunction

Why This Matters in Dentistry

- Dental infections (e.g. **spreading odontogenic infections**, deep neck space infections) can progress to sepsis
- Patients may present initially to dental services
- **Early recognition and rapid escalation save lives**
- Dental teams are expected to **recognise and escalate sepsis**, not provide definitive treatment[41]

Signs and Symptoms of Sepsis (Adults)

High-Risk Features ("Red Flags")

- New **altered mental state** (confusion, slurred speech)
- **Hypotension**
- **Tachycardia**
- **Tachypnoea**
- Oxygen saturation **below normal**
- **Low urine output**
- Pale, cold, clammy, or mottled skin
- Loss of consciousness

Other Features

- Fever **or** hypothermia
- Muscle aches
- Dizziness or syncope
- Nausea and vomiting

Important:
Normal temperature or absence of fever **does not exclude sepsis.**

Management in a Dental Practice

(Recognition and Escalation Only)

Immediate Actions – ABCDE Approach

1. **Stop dental treatment immediately**
2. **Call 999 or 112**
   - Clearly state: **"Suspected sepsis / septic shock"**
3. **Position the patient**
   - Supine if hypotensive
4. **Administer high-flow oxygen**
   - Target SpO_2:
     - **94–98%** (most adults)
     - **88–92%** (known COPD)
5. **Monitor vital signs continuously**
6. **Prepare for urgent transfer to hospital**

What NOT to Do in a Dental Practice

- Do **not** attempt IV fluid resuscitation
- Do **not** administer IV antibiotics
- Do **not** delay hospital transfer.

Hospital-based interventions include:

- IV fluids (e.g. 30 mL/kg)
- Vasopressors (e.g. noradrenaline)
- Blood cultures
- Lactate measurement
- IV antibiotics

These are **outside the scope of dental practice** and must not delay escalation[4041].

Key Learning Points

- Sepsis is a **medical emergency**
- Septic shock represents **circulatory failure**
- Dental teams must:
  - Recognise red-flag features
  - Use ABCDE assessment
  - Provide oxygen
  - Escalate **immediately**

- **Early recognition saves lives**

References

39. NICE. *Sepsis: Recognition, Diagnosis and Early Management (NG51)*
40. Singer M et al. *The Third International Consensus Definitions for Sepsis and Septic Shock (Sepsis-3)*
41. UK Sepsis Trust. *Sepsis Recognition and Management for Primary Care and Dental Teams*

Glossary

ABCDE / DRABCDE – Structured emergency assessment: Danger, Response, Airway, Breathing, Circulation, Disability, Exposure.

AED – Automated External Defibrillator.

Anaphylaxis – Rapid, life-threatening allergic reaction affecting airway, breathing, and circulation.

Buccal – Medication administered between cheek and gum.

CPR – Cardiopulmonary Resuscitation.

DNACPR – Do Not Attempt Cardiopulmonary Resuscitation.

Hypoglycaemia – Blood glucose <4.0 mmol/L.

IM – Intramuscular injection.

NEWS2 – National Early Warning Score.

PEA – Pulseless Electrical Activity.

ROSC – Return of Spontaneous Circulation.

SBAR – Situation, Background, Assessment, Recommendation.

Sepsis – Life-threatening organ dysfunction from dysregulated infection response.

SpO$_2$ – Peripheral oxygen saturation.

VF / VT – Ventricular fibrillation / ventricular tachycardia.

Index

BIBLIOGRAPHY

Statutory, Regulatory, and Professional Guidance

Care Quality Commission (CQC) (2014). *Regulation 12: Safe Care and Treatment.*
Department of Health and Social Care (2013). *HTM 01-05: Decontamination in Primary Care Dental Practices.*
General Dental Council (2024). *Standards for the Dental Team and Scope of Practice.*
Health and Social Care Act 2008 (Regulated Activities) Regulations 2014.
Human Medicines Regulations 2012.
Mental Capacity Act 2005 and Code of Practice.

Resuscitation and Emergency Care

European Resuscitation Council (2021). *ERC Guidelines for Resuscitation.*
Resuscitation Council UK (2015). *Safer Handling During Resuscitation in Healthcare Settings.*
Resuscitation Council UK (2021). *Adult Basic Life Support Guidelines.*
Resuscitation Council UK (2021). *Paediatric Basic Life Support Guidelines.*
Resuscitation Council UK (2021). *Medical Emergencies and Resuscitation Standards for Clinical Practice.*
Resuscitation Council UK (2021). *Defibrillation and Automated External Defibrillators.*

Cardiovascular and Cardiac Arrest

NICE (2007). *CG50: Acutely Ill Adults in Hospital.*
NICE (2013). *CG167: Myocardial Infarction with ST-Segment Elevation.*
Nolan, J.P., Smith, G.B., et al. (2014). 'Incidence and outcome of in-hospital cardiac arrest in the UK', *Resuscitation*, 85(8), pp. 987–992.
Vogel, B., Claessen, B.E., Arnold, S.V., et al. (2019). 'ST-segment elevation myocardial infarction', *Nature Reviews Disease Primers*, 5(1), 39.

Infection Prevention and Safety

UK Health Security Agency (2023). *National Infection Prevention and Control Manual*.
Public Health England (2016). *Dental Unit Waterlines: Advice on Infection Control*.
Health and Safety Executive (2013). *Safe Use and Disposal of Sharps*.
Health and Safety Executive (2018). *Safe Use of Compressed Gas Cylinders*.

Airway, Breathing, and Choking

Soar, J. and Nolan, J.P. (2013). 'Airway management in cardiopulmonary resuscitation', *Current Opinion in Critical Care*, 19(3), pp. 181–187.
Walls, R.M. and Murphy, M.F. (eds.) (2012). *Manual of Emergency Airway Management*, 4th ed. Philadelphia: Wolters Kluwer.
Office for National Statistics (2017). *Deaths Registered in England and Wales*.
NHS (2024). *Choking*. Available at: www.nhs.uk

Medical Emergencies

Asthma UK (2024). *Asthma Facts and Statistics*.
British National Formulary (2025). *BNF 89*. London: Pharmaceutical Press.
British Thoracic Society (2017). *Guideline for Oxygen Use in Adults in Healthcare and Emergency Settings*.
European Society of Cardiology (2009). *Guidelines for the Diagnosis and Management of Syncope*.
Gardner, W.N. (2003). 'Hyperventilation: A practical guide', *Medicine*, 31(11), pp. 7–8.
Joint British Diabetes Societies (JBDS) (2021). *The Hospital Management of Hypoglycaemia*.
NICE (2016). *NG51: Sepsis*.
NICE (2019). *NG136: Hypertension in Adults*.
NICE (2018). *NG115: COPD*.
NICE (2015). *NG17 / NG18: Diabetes*.

Singer, M., Deutschman, C.S., Seymour, C.W., et al. (2016). 'The Third International Consensus Definitions for Sepsis and Septic Shock (Sepsis-3)', *JAMA*, 315(8), pp. 801–810.

UK Sepsis Trust (2024). *Sepsis Recognition Tools for Primary Care.*

World Health Organization (2023). *Emergency Care Systems Framework.*

Medicines Law and Governance

GOV.UK (2025). *Rules for the Sale, Supply and Administration of Medicines.*

NHS England (2024). *Human Medicines (Amendments Relating to Dental Professionals).*

Scottish Dental Clinical Effectiveness Programme (SDCEP). *Drug Prescribing for Dentistry.*

www.ingramcontent.com/pod-product-compliance
Lightning Source LLC
Chambersburg PA
CBHW040853210326
41597CB00029B/4832